Brain Fables

Brain Fables

The Hidden History of Neurodegenerative Diseases and a Blueprint to Conquer Them

Alberto Espay
Professor of Neurology

Benjamin Stecher
Patient Advocate & Consultant

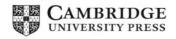
CAMBRIDGE
UNIVERSITY PRESS

CAMBRIDGE
UNIVERSITY PRESS

University Printing House, Cambridge CB2 8BS, United Kingdom

One Liberty Plaza, 20th Floor, New York, NY 10006, USA

477 Williamstown Road, Port Melbourne, VIC 3207, Australia

314–321, 3rd Floor, Plot 3, Splendor Forum, Jasola District Centre, New Delhi – 110025, India

79 Anson Road, #06–04/06, Singapore 079906

Cambridge University Press is part of the University of Cambridge.

It furthers the University's mission by disseminating knowledge in the pursuit of education, learning, and research at the highest international levels of excellence.

www.cambridge.org
Information on this title: www.cambridge.org/9781108744621
DOI: 10.1017/9781108888202

First published 2020

Printed in the United Kingdom by TJ International Ltd, Padstow Cornwall

A catalogue record for this publication is available from the British Library.

Library of Congress Cataloging-in-Publication Data
Names: Espay, Alberto J., author. | Stecher, Benjamin, author.
Title: Brain fables : the hidden history of neurodegenerative diseases and a blueprint to conquer them / Alberto Espay, University of Cincinnati, Benjamin Stecher, Educational Consultant & Healthcare Advocate.
Description: Cambridge, United Kingdom ; New York, NY : Cambridge University Press, [2020]
Identifiers: LCCN 2020004122 | ISBN 9781108744621 (paperback) | ISBN 9781108888202 (epub)
Subjects: LCSH: Nervous system – Degeneration.
Classification: LCC RC365 .E87 2020 | DDC 616.8–dc23
LC record available at https://lccn.loc.gov/2020004122

ISBN 978-1-108-74462-1 Paperback

....

For everyone living with a neurodegenerative disorder, for their caregivers and for the advocacy groups working to build a better tomorrow.

And for all those at the bedside and in the laboratory reconfiguring the war against brain aging and fine tuning its weaponry.

Contents

Preface 1 – The Question

Three years ago, the patriarch of a Cincinnati-based philanthropic foundation and patient of mine living with Parkinson's disease approached me with a question: If I had unlimited funding, how would I change the way we study and treat Parkinson's disease?

This was an unusual request. All funding for research is limited, which restricts the scope of the questions we can ask. As a practicing physician and clinical researcher, I have been trained to look for the most efficient way to answer whatever question I am investigating. This is the hypothesis-driven method of scientific inquiry, which allows us to answer small problems in a defined period of time with a finite set of resources. It also dictates that experiments should be based on accumulated data and on predictions of what might reasonably happen to a phenomenon or behavior after a given intervention. This is an important hinge around which medical science revolves. All experiments to date have been artifacts of funding restrictions in medical research and a homage to the idea that "fishing expeditions" are not good science. We *should know* what we are looking for.

For the last 15 years, neurologists working to answer questions about Parkinson's disease have lived in two different, mutually exclusive universes. Beginning in 2004,[1] we began accepting that Parkinson's disease may be an umbrella term for a spectrum of disorders, each with different symptoms, range of severity, and varying responses to treatments. The other universe is shaped by our belief that those variations are part of the same disease. Despite all the differences we see in our patients, we can target the disease as if it were one phenomenon. By searching for common threads, we tell ourselves, we will one day discover one or two biomarkers[1] that capture the complex biology of Parkinson's disease – and use them to develop therapies to slow disease progression in everyone with the disease.

At about the time of the philanthropist's request, a dear colleague and friend from Buenos Aires, Dr. Emilia Gatto, invited me to give a lecture she titled "Revision of the definition of Parkinson disease" for a symposium sponsored by the Pan-American Section of the International Parkinson and Movement Disorders Society, in March 2015. Just before, the Society's Task Force on the Definition of Parkinson's Disease had released revised criteria for diagnosing Parkinson's.[2] Emilia asked me to discuss the differences between the new and old versions of the clinical criteria for Parkinson's disease, but also encouraged me to critically assess the extent to which the changes would enable us to develop better symptomatic strategies and test new therapies to slow disease progression.

As I prepared the lecture on the "Redefinition of Parkinson's criteria" and thought more about the question posed by my patient, I found myself working on two parallel tracks that were not converging. What if our understanding of Parkinson's disease is also impeding our ability to find cures? Could it be that generating hypotheses based on what we think we know, along with our rigid funding models, is making it nearly impossible to find what we really need to know? After all, many of the most important scientific discoveries have come

---

[1] Biomarkers are any measurable indication of the presence or severity of a particular disease. One of the best examples is the monitoring of blood-glucose levels in diabetics. Development of biomarkers are critical for the development of new and improved therapies.

from dogged examination of the unknown, without preconceived hypotheses or restrictive lines of questioning.

This led me to perform a review of the data we were collecting in an ongoing biomarker development program funded by the Michael J. Fox Foundation called the Parkinson's Progression Markers Initiative (PPMI). This is the largest and most expensive study ever attempted to uncover biomarkers of Parkinson's disease. That analysis, as we will discuss in the book, led us to question the very foundations of this and similar programs.[3] By mid 2018, with two papers published, and a third on the way, challenging a central tenet of Parkinson's and Alzheimer's diseases (the causal role of aggregates of protein, alpha-synuclein in the case of Parkinson's and beta-amyloid and tau in the case of Alzheimer's),[4] I decided to reach out beyond my circle of neurologists. I contacted a *New York Times* journalist who had just published the article, "Scientists Racing to Cure Alzheimer's." That piece fit within the classic story line: undesirable proteins fill the brain of Parkinson's and Alzheimer's, and many treatments to clean them up are just within reach. In an email, I asked her if she would be interested in writing about "the other side." She replied, tersely: "Thanks for writing. You make a powerful case for biomarkers, but it is not clear that there are good biomarkers yet for Parkinson's disease. So, it does not seem to be a story for us at this time."

That statement became the spark that set this book in motion. She was correct, I had no biomarkers to trumpet. What I failed to convey to her was that the reason we had no biomarkers, and the way we were looking for them, *was the story*.

Neurodegenerative diseases do not exist. All are labels neurologists created before we had the insight and tools needed to accurately define them. So long as we cling to them, we will never find what we are looking for.

Time has come to put an end to these fables.

Alberto J. Espay, MD, MSc, FAAN

Preface 2 – Enter Patient

At roughly the same time that Alberto was approached by his patient philanthropist in Cincinnati with the question that would lead him to want to write this book, I was on the other side of the planet coming to grips with a similar conundrum.

In November 2013, I was diagnosed with Parkinson's disease. I was a 29-year-old kid doing quite well for myself as a managing director of an education company in Shanghai when I got the news.

I didn't know anything about the disease at the time. I had no family history of Parkinson's, and I hadn't even heard of anyone with it outside of Muhammed Ali and Michael J. Fox. I went and found a clip of Ali lighting the torch at the 1996 Summer Olympics in Atlanta and intently watched his quivering hands as he lit that giant flame. Most people probably look at that moment as a defiant act of courage from this great man who had conquered the world and not let anything stop him from getting what he wanted out of life; not Joe Frazier, not the United States Government, and not Parkinson's disease. But what I saw when I looked back at that film was the future I was now doomed to live: hands trembling, frozen expression on my face, barely able to walk properly, probably reliant on a myriad of different pills just to make an appearance.

It's not easy figuring out how to move on with life as a young man faced with that kind of fate. Our healthcare systems aren't much help. Patients typically get 20 minutes every six months with their neurologist, just enough time to go through an awkward series of motor tests and questions that supposedly say something important about our disease before a prescription is written and token words of encouragement exchanged.

So where to go? Who to talk to? At any other time in history there would be nothing that anyone on Earth could do. But we live in remarkable times, I soon realized I had more resources at my disposal than any king or emperor had ever dreamed.

To the Internet I went. There I found people all over the world working diligently to fix what was ailing me. It was strange and confusing at first. The last biology class I took was in tenth grade, but over time I got used to the vocabulary and started being able to make sense of the papers I was reading. I soon found myself enthralled by the puzzle that is the human brain and why certain parts of it degenerate faster in some than others.

Before long, just reading the papers was not enough. I wanted to know what was happening at the bleeding edge of research, what was in the pipeline, and what I could do to help speed things up. As my symptoms progressed, I also became keenly aware that this puzzle was going to be too important to me to simply leave to others to figure out.

Which brings me to that moment in time three years ago when, as Alberto was toiling with how to reconcile the request from his patient benefactor with the newfound understanding he was developing about the search for biomarkers, I decided to leave my career in China behind and dive head first into this field for an accelerated course of study.

I have since spent my time touring some of the top biomedical labs on the planet and meeting with hundreds of the best physicians and scientists in the field. (And, as any good millennial would, I started a website (tmrwedition.com) where, as of this writing, I have interviewed over 80 world experts on the subject.)

Parkinson's sucks, but I wouldn't trade these last few years for anything. The information age and this disease have gotten my foot in the door into places I would otherwise never have been. It also gave me the chance to observe science in action as it pushes forward a frontier of knowledge. I have learned more along the way about the brain, biology, and disease than I ever thought possible. However, I have also learned that medical science is not quite what I thought it was.

For most of my life I was a passive consumer of science. I'd read a few articles and popular science books here and there, and generally took as gospel most of what was acknowledged to be scientific consensus. From the outside, science looks like the ultimate storehouse of credibility from which all that we know about the world emerges fully formed. However, for the last few years I have have been able to enter that house and browse the section labeled "Neurology and Neuroscience – Subsection: Parkinsonisms." At first glance it appeared relatively neat and tidy. But having now read through many of its volumes, and having met most of its living authors (and even contributed a few pages myself), I see that many of its volumes have been filled by narratives we created that might be blurring our ability to distinguish truth from fiction, slowing us down in our attempts to effectively treat these diseases.

I now find myself in a rather unique position. On the one hand, I'm a patient patiently waiting for new therapies to come online. On the other, I also now get flown around the world to attend meetings and conferences about this disease and share my insight into what we should be doing next.

The question that now drives me, which I think is fundamentally the same one Alberto faces, is how to do the most good with this position I find myself in? What direction should we be going in? How can I leverage my influence to accelerate the development of better therapies for myself, for the 7 million to 10 million others around the world living with this condition, and the millions more yet to be diagnosed?

For me, this book is an attempt to answer that question, to lay out some of the most important lessons I have learned from all the people I have interacted with along the way, and to help shed some light on a new way of thinking which I believe may be our best hope to one day finally putting an end to degenerative brain diseases.

Benjamin Stecher

Acknowledgements

A Note of Gratitude from Alberto Espay

This book wouldn't be possible if it were not for the dedication of many people to the multifaceted task of rethinking neurodegenerative diseases, particularly our friends and colleagues at the University of Cincinnati (Dr. Brett Kissela, Dr. Joe Broderick, Dr. Dan Woo, and Dr. Andrew Duker), the University of Toronto (Dr. Anthony Lang, Dr. Alfonso Fasano, and Dr. Lorraine Kalia), and the Parkinson Study Group (Dr. Michael Schwarzschild, Dr. Hubert Fernandez, Dr. David Simon, Dr. Carlie Tanner, Dr. Karl Kieburtz, Dr. Jim Leverenz, and Dr. David Standaert).

I owe a big deal of gratitude to the Gardner Family in Cincinnati whose foundation was instrumental in the creation of the James J. and Joan A. Gardner Family Center for Parkinson's Disease and Movement Disorders at the University of Cincinnati. Gary and Peggy Johns, Linda Mueller and the late Tom Mueller, and their dynamic "G3s", Adam, Eric, and Jonathan as well as Peggy, Lori and Spencer Gardner. I am also thankful to Bobby and Katie Lawrence, Jerry and Sandy Wuest, Dave and Linda Armstrong, David Wyse, and so many others from our community of patients and patient advocates who have contributed in unique ways to the fabric of our success.

Special recognition goes to the members of the Cincinnati Cohort Biomarker Program (CCBP), now fully active at the University of Cincinnati. They have been laser-focused on enacting the blueprint proposed in this book despite the many grueling tasks required to do so. The current CCBP workforce is composed of Dawn Skirpan (program manager), Dr. Luca Marsili, Dr. Andrea Sturchio, Elizabeth Keeling, Nathan Gregor, Cynthia Spikes, Deepa Agrawal Bajaj, Kevin Duque, Hussein Abdelghany, and Erin Neefus.

Finally, I thank the Farmer Family Foundation for giving me the gift of dreaming by posing their fundamental questions. I am also indebted to Nick Dunton, Anna Whiting, and Camille Lee-Own, from Cambridge University Press, for their encouragement to publish this book and the thoughtful feedback provided along the way; Marcia Hartsock and Tonya Hines, for their compelling medical illustrations, and Luisa Jung, for the cover art and introductory chapter illustrations; Peggy A'Hearn, for her expert liaison of our work with prospective funders through the University of Cincinnati Foundation; Cindy Starr, journalist with a neuroscientist mindset and a global vision of neurology, for the careful proofreading and editing; Jo Tyszka, for equally masterful postsubmission copyediting; and Kristy Espay, my soul mate, who spent many nights helping me refine these ideas for the public.

Special Thanks from Benjamin Stecher

My journey that led to this book connected me to so many people that have at one point or another taken the time to guide me through this complex maze. Though I wish I never had reason to get to know you all, I am glad I did.

My sincere gratitude to: Dr. Alfonso Fasano, Dr. Hilal A. Lashuel, Dr. Gerold Riempp, Sara Riggare, Mariette Robijn, Martin Taylor, Gina Lupino, Dr. Simon Stott, Hugh Johnston, Sherrie Gould, Dr. Ziv Gan-Or, Dr. Tilo Kunath, Dr. Heidi McBride, Dr. Patrik Brundin, Dr. Peter Lansbury, Dr. Hyunsoo Shawn Je, Dr. Karen Raphael, Harry McMurtry, Dr. Jon Stamford, Helen Matthews, Lisa Vanderburg, Gaynor Edwards, Bob Dulich, Omotola Thomas, Dr. Anthony E. Lang, Dr. Jeanne Loring, David Ashford Jones, Jonathan Silverstein, Dr. Markus Britschgi, Dr. Joseph Geraci, Dr. Julie Andersen, Dr. Gaia Skibinksi, Dr. Edward A. Fon, Ofer Nemirovsky, Heather Kennedy, Dr. Julian and Fran Lo, Annabel Seyller, Dr. Soania Mathur, Matt Ackerman, Alex Reed, Dr. Leonard Sokol, Dr. Jon Palfreman, Dr. Shane Liddelow, Lev and Galina Leytes, Dr. Andrew Lees, Dr. Kalpana Merchant, Dr. Alice Chen-Plotkin, Dr. Lorraine Kalia, Nenad Bach, Dr. Roger Barker, Dr. Richard Wyse, Dr. Jeffrey Kordower, and Dr. Megan Duffy.

Thank you as well to all the family and friends that have lent their support along the way. And a final thank you to the two people who I owe everything to, my parents.

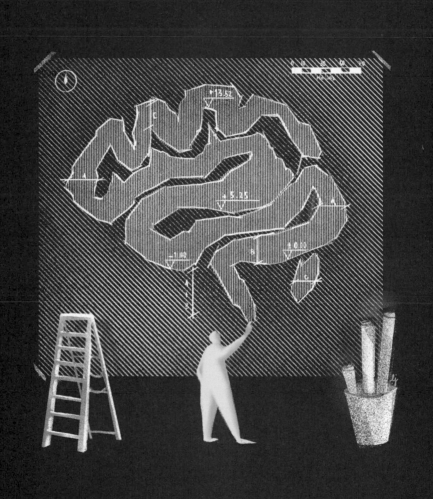

The Shaky Six and the "Second Reality"

The crucial importance of cognitive dissonance. Humans have an amazing capacity to believe in contradictory things. For example, to believe in an omnipotent and benevolent God, but somehow excuse Him from all the suffering in the world. Or our ability to believe from the standpoint of law that humans are equal and have free will and from biology that humans are just organic machines. Our medical system and our legal system are built on contradictory assumptions. Yet we somehow live with this contradiction.

Yuval Noah Harari, in answer to "What's the most misunderstood fact about the history of our species?", posed by Arik Gabbai, Smithsonian, February 2015

In *Sapiens,* Yuval Noah Harari argues that humankind's greatest invention is our ability to create and believe fictions. While all other animals communicate realities with which they interact, humans create a separate layer of subjective, interpretative realities. The fiction most universally embraced today is money. "Dollar bills have absolutely no value except in our collective imagination, but everybody believes in the dollar bill," says Harari.

Harari goes on to state that humans have been living in a dual reality. "On the one hand, the *objective reality* of rivers, trees, and lions; and on the other hand, the *imagined reality* of gods, nations, and corporations."

In medicine, humans have also created two realities.

Clinicians describe what they see, an *objective* reality, but the medical community then tries to explain and give meaning to what they see, creating a second, *imagined* reality. When a sufficient collection of objective realities are viewed, patterns emerge and an idea of a disease starts to form. The validity of the second, imagined reality gets verified by the accumulation and replication of the emergent patterns. When this second reality spreads far enough, it becomes the accepted reality. In so doing, it also becomes resistant to any evidence to the contrary.

In 1817 Dr. James Parkinson published his interpretations of physical features shared by three patients he examined in his office and three other individuals he observed on the streets of London: tremor in one hand, slowness of movement, stiffness, stooped posture, and difficulties with walking and balance. He proposed the term *paralysis agitans* to describe those who were affected. Parkinson was the epitome of the astute clinician living in an era in which observation was the greatest instrument of medicine. His detailed notes meticulously described the collection of abnormalities he observed. When read today, his monograph, *An Essay on the Shaking Palsy,* remains a remarkably elegant and vivid piece of neurology.

So slight and nearly imperceptible are the first inroads of this malady, and so extremely slow its progress, that it rarely happens, that the patient can form any recollection of the precise period of its commencement. The first symptoms perceived are a slight sense of weakness, with a proneness to trembling in some particular part; sometimes in the head, but most commonly in one of the hands and arms. These symptoms gradually increase in the part first affected; and at an uncertain period, but seldom in less than twelve months or more, the morbid influence is felt in some other part. Thus assuming one of the hands and arms to be first attacked, the other, at this period becomes similarly affected. After a few more months the patient is found to be less strict than usual in preserving an upright posture: this being most observable whilst walking, but sometimes whilst sitting or standing.

[...]

But as the malady proceeds, even this temporary mitigation of suffering from the agitation of the limbs is denied. The propensity to lean forward becomes invincible, and the patient is thereby forced to step on the toes and fore part of the feet, whilst the upper part of the body is thrown so far forward as to render it difficult to avoid falling on the face. In some cases, when this state of the malady is attained, the patient can no longer exercise himself by walking in his usual manner, but is thrown on the toes and forepart of the feet; being, at the same time, irresistibly impelled to take much quicker and shorter steps, and thereby to adopt unwillingly a running pace. In some cases it is found necessary entirely to substitute running for walking; since otherwise the patient, on proceeding only a very few paces, would inevitably fall.

An Essay on the Shaking Palsy, by James Parkinson, monograph
published by Sherwood, Neely, and Jones (London, 1817)

In 1861 the famous French neurologist Dr. Jean-Martin Charcot recognized and extended Parkinson's observations on the *paralysis agitans*, but emphasized that patients were neither markedly weakened nor necessarily plagued with tremor.[5] Nevertheless, Charcot suggested applying to this cluster of neurological difficulties the name "Parkinson's disease" in honor of Parkinson's seminal description.

The most important elements of the "second, imagined reality" was completed nearly a century after the Shaky Six from London came to the attention of the medical field. In 1912 a German neurologist, Dr. Friedrich Heinrich Lewy, working on the brains of individuals who had died with the symptoms Parkinson identified, found unusual clumps of proteins inside neurons in certain parts of the brain.[6]

The *corps de Lewy* – or Lewy bodies, as coined by Dr. Konstantin Trétiakoff, a Russian neuropathologist – provided the first evidence of clinical observations converging with brain tissue observations, validating the label Parkinson's *disease* (Figure 1). This was to become the "clinico-pathologic" model enshrined by nineteenth-century physicians. The recognition of specific brain proteins at autopsy became the gold standard for definitive diagnoses of all diseases of brain aging. With the proliferation of new staining methods and advances in microscopy, the type of proteins to be identified during postmortem studies was to grow in diversity in the twentieth century.

As the same type of protein was observed in brains from people who died with or without dementia, with or without tremor, with rapid or slow progression, Parkinson's and other age-related diseases cemented themselves as heterogeneous, but ultimately single diseases.

An easily overlooked implication is that neuropathologists became the arbiters of diseases and disease classifications. Clinicians could achieve "possible" or, at best, "probable" categories of diagnostic certainty when examining a patient, but they couldn't be "definitive." The elevation of the diagnostic certainty to "definitive" was reserved for the outcome of microscopic examination of brain tissue after death.

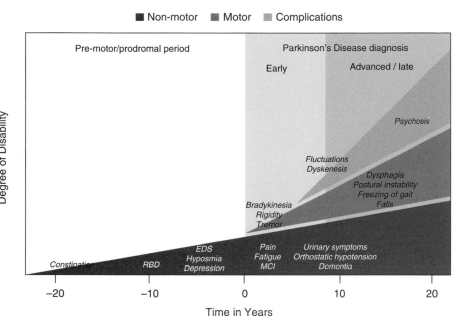

Figure 1 A heterogeneous disease. The "confirmation" of Parkinson's disease by Lewy bodies identified at autopsy increased the spectrum of manifestations thought to represent the same disease. This diagram depicts the range of motor and non-motor features believed to arise from Lewy bodies at "Time 0," defined arbitrarily as the time when the first motor symptom appears, which is when the disease becomes recognizable to physicians and can be diagnosed at the bedside (adapted by Marcia Hartsock, from Lang and Kalia, *Lancet* 2015;386 (9996): 896–912). RBD: REM sleep behavior disorder; EDS: excessive daytime sleepiness; MCI: mild cognitive impairment.

The importance of the study of brain tissue in the classifications of diseases (*nosology*, in the jargon of medicine) was eventually going to give birth to the concept that neurodegenerative diseases, or diseases of abnormal brain aging, were "proteinopathies." According to this model, I can tell you what disease you have if you tell me what proteins your brain accumulates. (More on these proteins and what they mean in Chapter 5.)

One final wrinkle worth considering. When James Parkinson was hard at work describing the Shaky Six, he probably thought he was describing a set of features that were common to selected individuals and distinguishable from other diseases. If we could ask him today, he might say that he was describing a syndrome, a collection of discrete symptoms and signs that formed a clinical pattern. It is unlikely he was proposing a distinct molecular entity.[1]

Yet 200 years later we celebrate James Parkinson because the field still sees in his work something beyond what he intended. In this narrative we have embraced, he was describing

---

[1] If biological or molecular abnormalities affect function, they produce symptoms. Conversely, symptoms cannot be expected to reflect a specific biological or molecular abnormality. Most symptoms are non-specific manifestations of many abnormalities. A *disease* is considered a reflection of specific biological/molecular abnormalities, often yielding a set of heterogeneous symptoms. A syndrome is defined as a collection of diseases and, as such, cannot be specific to any biological/molecular abnormalities.

not just a syndrome but a biological and molecular construct – which, we anticipate we are on the brink of finally demonstrating. In the chapters to come, we shall uncover the pitfalls of this deeply ingrained "second reality."

Commentary – What Is and What Isn't

The universe seeks equilibriums; it prefers to disperse energy, disrupt organization, and maximize chaos. Life is designed to combat these forces. We slow down reactions, concentrate matter, and organize chemicals into compartments; we sort laundry on Wednesdays. "It sometimes seems as if curbing entropy is our quixotic purpose in the universe," James Gleick wrote. We live in the loopholes of natural laws, seeking extensions, exceptions and excuses. The laws of nature still mark the outer boundaries of permissibility – but life, in all its idiosyncratic, mad weirdness, flourishes by reading between the lines.

Siddhartha Mukherjee, The Gene: An Intimate History

The most challenging part of my diagnosis has been trying to figure out what and who to believe in. Not a week goes by that a family member or friend doesn't send me news of some therapy or supplement that supposedly does wonders for Parkinson's. Early on I followed up on every one. Some took me down some very bizarre rabbit holes. Almost all ended in disappointment.

Over time I became better at sniffing out which were worth exploring and which I could ignore. One of the few good things about Parkinson's is that it tends to progress slowly, giving most who get it enough time to come to a pretty good understanding of it. But it is a long slow road to comprehension, one born out of fear, frustration, and endless trial-and-error.

Here is one such rabbit hole I fell into: On a trip back to China in December of 2016, a friend brought me to a lecture hall in Shanghai to meet a renowned practitioner of traditional Chinese medicine (TCM). Going in I was more than a little skeptical, but I promised to be open minded enough to see what, if any, insight this doctor might have for me. What I didn't know when I walked in was that I would be interrupting her class so that she could use me as a live guinea pig for her techniques, and as a foreign prop to impress her audience.

She started by having me sit in a chair while she passed her hand over me to examine my qi (a force that can be harnessed and used as a measure of one's vitality). Afterwards she took out a small container of seeds and started taping them to my ear while the class gathered around. According to some branches of TCM, the entire body can be mapped to pressure points on the ears, hands or feet, and certain seeds can trigger neurological connections between the various parts of the body that stimulate healing. So, for about 20 minutes I sat there as dozens of tiny seeds were pressed into both ears.

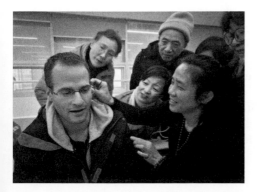

Figure 2 "The Experiment." Class gathers for a live demonstra-tion of the therapeutic benefits of a bold new technique for people with Parkinson's.

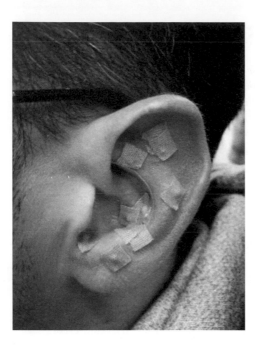

Figure 3 "The Aftermath." A dozen or so tiny seeds, renowned for their healing powers, were pressed onto my ear...still awaiting supposed benefit.

She then took out a hand-carved wooden comb and started delivering vibrating pulses against my scalp. She did this for about 10 minutes while she explained the mystical powers of the wood it was carved from. I could hear the hushed words from those in attendance: "Look, he's getting better" and "wow, it's working." I only felt the tremor-like scrapes of the comb against my head.

Afterwards she gave me the comb and a beaded wooden bracelet to wear and told me to walk West for one hour a day until I was cured.

Yuval Noah Harari has been one of the most helpful guides I have had in helping me separate fact from fiction. He has a knack for cutting through the noise and getting right to the most important details. From him I learned that when trying to understand a truth of our world, you must remove any form of narrative. All stories are the creation of our subjective experiences, and often they blur the line between what is and what isn't. He seems to apply this to everything he studies, from our mythologies and religions, to money and nations. I wonder if he would say the same thing about biomedical science?

At a fundamental level there are enormous gaps between what we know about our biology and what there is to know. We know there are 20 organic compounds called amino acids that make up everything we think of as life. But how they assemble into all the pieces that make us who we are, and how those pieces interact with one another, is, for the most part, a black box. This makes it very difficult for us to properly intervene when things go wrong.

This was explained to me in an interview I did with Dario Alessi, professor at the University of Dundee in Scotland and one of the most revered biochemists in the field:

Generally, I think we understand less than 1/10,000 of all that there is to understand in biology. We know virtually nothing about how biology is controlled and how it works.

We have 20,000+ genes, each with many different variants, which are all expressed at different levels, in different ways, in different cells. They probably make hundreds of thousands of RNA molecules and millions of forms of proteins that get modified in a number of ways. All of these things interact and form the various parts of the cell. Also, as you interact with your environment and consume energy, DNA accumulates damage that also affects how cells function. All of this is like a big boiling pot with millions of things thrown in; you can't really understand it.

Posted September 18, 2018, *tmrwedition.com*

So, what do humans do when they try to make sense of something that they don't really understand? They make it up, filling in the gaps with stories about what we think is happening. Our most probable stories now get called hypotheses, which we then test to see if we can accept as truth. In medicine those "truths" lead to potential treatments which we push through the clinical trial process hoping some make it out the other side.

As Dario went on to say in that interview: "There isn't a lot of funding to do the fundamental research on one gene or one protein that would be needed to really understand these things. You could spend your whole life studying one protein, but getting the funding to do that is hard. Funding bodies want us to solve diseases and work with companies to figure out shortcuts that can be made into a drug. But we don't have the fundamental basis needed to really solve these problems."

And therein lies the crux of this problem. How can we intervene in something we don't understand? How many of the pieces of this puzzle have we uncovered? How many more do we need to be able to purposefully intervene?

Here some would say: "But medical science is filled with stories of accidental break-throughs; maybe if we continue doing as we have done up till now we will stumble across a solution." As George Church, world-renowned geneticist and professor at Harvard University, put it in an interview with me, "We developed effective smallpox prevention back when we had close to zero understanding of virology and immunology." Sure, it is possible, but is that the strategy you would bet your life on?

Our Best Bets

So what is the field placing its bets on? What do the experts think we should be devoting our limited resources to? I wanted to find out, so I took a poll, asking many of the experts I know to list their top five disease-modifying targets for Parkinson's; 43 of them responded (Figure 4).

Of the 43 experts polled, 35 said that alpha-synuclein (*SNCA* is the name of the corresponding gene) represents our best target to modify the course of this disease. This wasn't really a surprise, one of my first interviews was with Jeffrey H. Kordower, an international authority on movement disorders and professor at Rush University, who

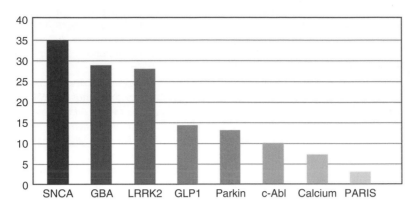

Figure 4 Unscientific survey of scientists. Experts were given a list of presumed genetic and molecular targets for therapeutic development and asked which ones they thought were most likely to succeed.

told me, "In terms of cures, I am for testing everything that modifies synuclein. I often say, synuclein now, synuclein forever."

At first this was comforting, a single misfolding protein seemed like a nice tidy explanation and a clear target to go after. Stop these clumps from forming, and we'll stop the disease. I dug a little deeper and saw that the evidence was pretty compelling. For one, families with a rare duplication or triplication of the *SNCA* gene have drastically higher rates of the disease. Additionally, autopsies revealed that the vast majority of people who have died with Parkinson's had these proteins aggregating in their brains. These pieces of evidence were enough to get alpha-synuclein labelled *pathogenic*, meaning the *cause* of disease.

But dig a little deeper and you start to see that there are a few holes in this theory. For one, despite a couple of decades of research into this misfolding protein, we still know very little about what the healthy version of it is supposed to do.

Kelvin Luk, a protein-folding expert at the University of Pennsylvania, which may be the world's leading center in the study of synuclein, explained to me, "We know that once this protein starts to misfold (that is, adopt an abnormal shape), it triggers a cascade of more misfolding. The cause for the initial misfolding is still a black box because we still know very little about the correct shape that alpha-synuclein should be in for it to function properly."

To me this seems like trying to fix a broken car radiator without even knowing what a radiator does or why it was there in the first place. At some point I started to question, if we know so little about this protein, why are we so sure that it is the cause of this disease?

I went back and reread an interview with Simon Stott, then a research associate at Cambridge University and now deputy director of research at the Cure Parkinson's Trust. "While I hope that it is a cause because we have all these clinical trials going on targeting it, I think the community needs to prepare itself that it isn't that simple. The brain is so complicated, I seriously doubt that it comes down to one protein. If it really was that simple, then we would probably be too simple to understand it."

The more I came to know about this disease, and the more I examined our failures of the past, the more I started to realize that time and time again we had fallen short because we believed that the problem was simpler than it really was. Yet almost every book ever written about the brain starts by marveling at its complexity, astounding readers with its hundred billion cells and the hundred trillion connections between them that together form the most sophisticated clump of matter in the known universe. How do we even begin to look for all the pieces needed to make sense of such a complicated puzzle, let alone decide that any one puzzle piece is responsible for things that go wrong?

What if, as Alberto will elaborate in the next chapter, we have been looking for pieces to a puzzle that doesn't even exist?

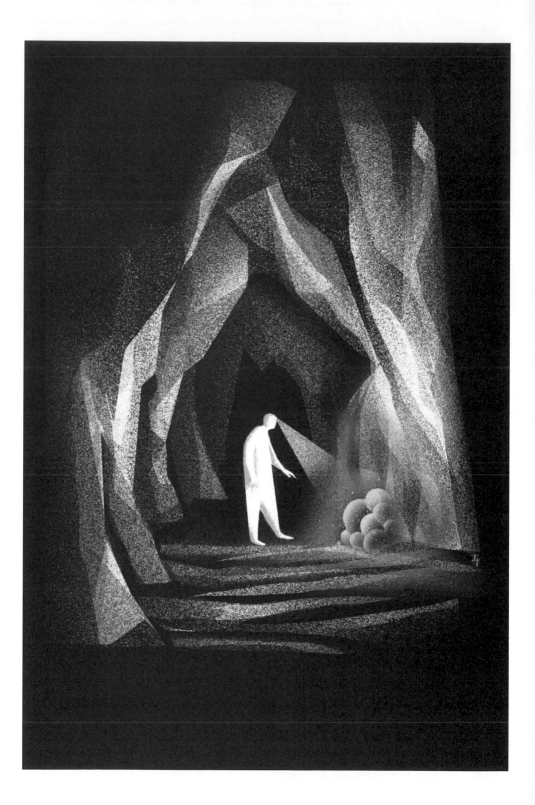

Pieces of a Puzzle?

Here were six patients whose symptoms modeled, down to the last detail, one of the major unsolved degenerative diseases of the aging brain.

J. W. Langston and J. P. Palfreman, The Case of the Frozen Addicts: How the Solution of a Medical Mystery Revolutionized the Understanding of Parkinson's Disease. *IOS Press,* 2014[7]

Levodopa is the closest thing we have to a miracle in modern medicine. When people with Parkinson's disease start treatment with this molecule and its dose is titrated to an optimal level, many symptoms vanish – at least for the duration of its therapeutic action. The effect on the overall function of a patient affected by Parkinson's symptoms is so marked that "response to levodopa" was enshrined as part of the clinical diagnosis of Parkinson's disease. Lack of or poor response to levodopa raises the concern that the patient might not have Parkinson's disease at all.

The story of how levodopa came into existence might be one of the most dramatic in all of neurology. The first milestone started with Arvid Carlsson, a Swedish pharmacologist who showed, in 1957, that levodopa restored mobility to a paralyzed rabbit. Carlsson demonstrated that reserpine (a drug used to induce paralysis in animal models) depleted the brain of dopamine, and that a reduction in dopamine is what reduces mobility. Levodopa could restore brain dopamine levels and normalize movement. These remarkable discoveries earned him the Nobel Prize in physiology and medicine (shared with Eric Kandel and Paul Greengard in 2000). Carlsson's work inspired the Austrian biochemist Oleh Hornykiewicz to quantify dopamine in the striatum, a part of the brain involved in the control of movement, using autopsy material from patients who had had Parkinson's disease. In 1960, he reported that marked depletion of dopamine in the striatum was common to people with Parkinson's disease. He went on to show that the more severe the loss of dopamine in the striatum, the worse the slowness and stiffness.

Since dopamine cannot enter the brain but must be generated from within, Hornykiewicz injected its precursor, levodopa, into 20 Parkinson's disease patients. This first act of brain dopamine replacement led to the first veritable *awakening*. Patients with stiffened, sluggish limbs and muffled voices limbered into full mobility, their arms and legs alive with agility they had not shown in years. This effect only lasted a few minutes, but left a tantalizing taste of what was to come.

At first, oral levodopa could not replicate the impact of the injectable form. It wasn't until 1967 when the Greek-American neurologist Dr. George Cotzias approached the problem with daring tenacity. With doses of levodopa anyone else would have considered ridiculously high, he showed a dramatic reversal of Parkinson's symptoms. He had worked

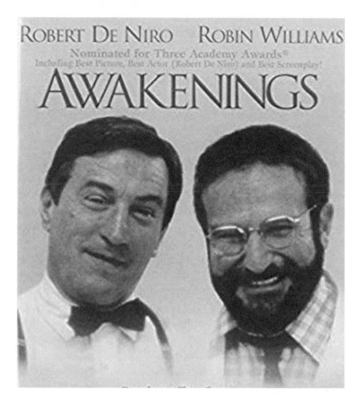

Figure 5 Awakenings is a 1990 American film based on Oliver Sacks' 1973 book of the same title. It tells the story of Dr. Malcolm Sayer (Robin Williams), who, in 1969, discovers the beneficial effects of levodopa and administers it to patients who survived the 1917–28 epidemic of encephalitis lethargica with a syndrome very similar to that of Parkinson's disease. Like other patients, Leonard Lowe (Robert De Niro) is literally *awakened* after decades of a catatonia-like state, including the drama of a life resumed after a long pause – and a glimpse of levodopa's shortcomings. The film was nominated for three Academy Awards.

on increasing his patients' dosage at slow increments, hoping that they would adapt to the nausea and vomiting levodopa brought with it. It would be made clear eventually that these gastrointestinal side effects were due to the transformation of levodopa into dopamine while still in the bloodstream, before levodopa could cross into the brain. The development of molecules that prevented that conversion, such as carbidopa and benserazide, enabled the delivery of levodopa without nausea and at a much lower dose. Levodopa was finally available, close to its present form, in 1975.

Levodopa became to Parkinson's what insulin was to diabetes. It helped restore the brain dopamine levels and temporarily relieved the restricted mobility dopamine deficiency created. Levodopa and, to a lesser extent other dopamine-enhancing treatments that followed, have been the closest thing we have to a miracle for many patients. Many at the time believed levodopa was the cure for Parkinson's (Figure 5). And because the effect was so pronounced across virtually all patients, it added weight to the notion that Parkinson's was one disease.

Let us summarize the narrative that has emerged: the disease is *suggested* by the presence of slowness of movements and stiffness, *supported* by a robust response to levodopa during life, and *confirmed* by the discovery of the Lewy pathology upon death.

This unified view of a disease was to be cemented by three additional discoveries: the finding in 1982 that a toxin, MPTP, could give rise to the clinical features of Parkinson's; the identification of alpha-synuclein in 1997 as *the* Parkinson's gene and the major constituent of the Lewy bodies; and the discovery that Lewy pathology could be detectable in the colon years before the onset of Parkinson's symptoms and might have a predictable pattern of progression. These last observations ultimately materialized into what came to be known as the Braak hypothesis in 2003.

MPTP

In July 1982, Dr. J William Langston, directing the neurology division at the Santa Clara Valley Medical Center in San Jose, California, received a call from his chief resident, Phil Ballard: "Dr. Langston, you have to come down here, I've never seen anything like it, and no one is sure what this patient has." Langston was initially reluctant to see George Carrillo, the man who was going to change not only his career but the entire direction of Parkinson's research.[7,8]

George Carrillo lay propped up in bed, staring vacantly, his mouth locked open and drooling, his arms frozen bent at his side. He could not speak. His zombie-like state caused the psychiatrists who first evaluated him to diagnose him with catatonic schizophrenia.

The documentation of the neurological examination showed very unusual features. After Langston held Carrillo's arms straight out and let them go, they stayed fixed in the position in which they were held, a phenomenon called "waxy flexibility." When Langston repetitively tapped Carrillo's forehead between the eyebrows, the blinking reflex would not habitutate; he kept on blinking, a sign referred to as the "Myerson's sign." When Langston asked Carrillo to forcefully close his eyes and then quickly open them, the eyelids would not separate quickly enough, instead they involuntarily closed for longer than desired, noted in the records as "eyelid apraxia." All of these neurological signs are today considered "red flags" against the diagnosis of Parkinson's disease; a neurologist with movement disorders training would not use the diagnostic label Parkinson's disease for these symptoms, especially given their rapid appearance. Nevertheless, Carrillo reminded Langston of the way advanced Parkinson's patients may have looked like before the advent of levodopa. And, in fact, when Carrillo was given levodopa, he experienced a marked and immediate "awakening." The conclusion was that Carrillo must have accrued a form of Parkinson's disease.

George Carrillo was the first of a total of six patients that Langston would come to know that exhibited a rapid onset of near-frozenness ultimately traced to a synthetic or "designer" form of heroin available in northern California. The painstaking work to explain the motionless state of these individuals led to the identification, in this heroin batch, of the toxin MPP+, derived from MPTP,[1] which was selectively toxic to the substantia nigra, the part of the midbrain most critical for the production of dopamine. The findings were published in *Science* in 1983, which became one of the most cited papers in the field of Parkinson's disease.[9] Langston held this discovery as a "tool to study nigrostriatal degeneration and ways to prevent it (...), *a human model of the animal model of the human disease.*"[8]

---

[1] MPTP stands for 1-methyl-4-phenyl-1,2,5,6-tetrahydropyridine, generated from the intravenous self-injection of the unusual synthetic heroin, which, by the enzyme monoamine oxidase B (MAO-B), turns into the neurotoxic cation MPP+, or 1-methyl-4-phenylpyridinium. MPTP selectively destroys the neurons of the substantia nigra pars compacta in the midbrain, the brain's major factory of dopamine.

That an environmental toxin could generate a disease so close to the real thing was soon regarded as support for the argument that selected environmental exposures were capable of bringing on Parkinson's disease. For instance, the herbicide paraquat, with toxic activity similar to that of MPTP, has been shown to increase the risk for Parkinson's disease.[10]

Mice "treated" with MPTP became the best established model of Parkinson's, yielding to date over 7,000 publications, and serving as the testing grounds for many disease mechanisms and interventions. Because the toxin affects the neurons that produce dopamine, MPTP-treated animals have been used to evaluate the effect of dopamine-enhancing therapies, some of which eventually became available to ameliorate symptoms of Parkinson's that come from low levels of dopamine.

However, this discovery might have done more to slow than to accelerate the development of disease-modifying therapies for Parkinson's. The rapid destruction of the substantia nigra by MPTP is very much unlike the slow, progressive neurodegeneration of this region and many others in the brains of individuals with Parkinson's disease. Despite the critical differences in the nature of the affected brain region, the tempo of progression, and the clinical picture, MPTP has remained the go-to model to glean insights into potential therapies. From its discovery all the way up to 2016, there have been over 500 published reports of compounds or therapies that were validated based on evidence from MPTP-treated animal models (Figure 6). All have failed to translate to the real disease.[2]

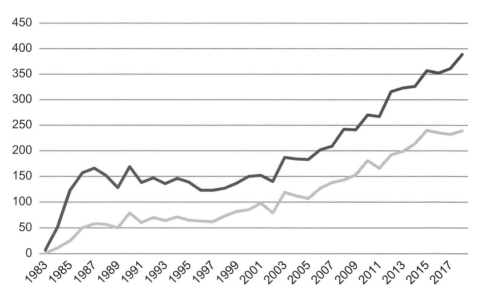

Figure 6 MPTP-related publications (Pubmed, 1983–2018). A total of 7,022 MPTP-related research projects (black line) have been published since the first report in 1983. Of those, 4,003 publications (gray line) are associated with the keywords "treatment" or "therapy." MPTP, 1-methyl-4-phenyl-1,2,3,6-tetrahydropyridine. Search terms: * 6-tetrahydropyridine"[Mesh] OR "MPTP Poisoning"[Mesh] OR mptp NOT (review or "Review" [Publication Type]) ^ 6-tetrahydropyridine"[Mesh] OR "MPTP Poisoning"[Mesh] OR mptp NOT (review or "Review" [Publication Type]) AND (treatment OR therapy). Analysis courtesy of Dr. Joaquin Vizcarra.

---

[2] Because of the enzyme MAO-B's role in converting MPTP into the toxic MPP+, which is deadly to substantia nigra neurons, MAO-B inhibitors (selegiline in the late 1980s; rasagiline in the late 2000s) were heavily studied as potentially disease-modifying treatments.

Alpha-synuclein Mutations

If the discovery of MPTP put the environment front and center as the likely *cause* of Parkinson's disease, the discoveries of rare families with Parkinson's, beginning in the late 1990s, would swing the research pendulum decisively toward genetics. Dr. Roger Duvoisin, Chair of Neurology at Rutgers New Jersey Medical School in New Brunswick (now Rutgers Robert Wood Johnson), encountered a patient with an extensive family history of Parkinson's disease in 1979. Along with Dr. Lawrence (Larry) Golbe, he embarked on a genealogical study of this family, as well as another from New York, and found that they all came from the same town, Contursi, in the Campagna region of southern Italy, near Salerno. Golbe expanded his study of the New Jersey and New York families to include two others from Contursi. In 1990 he and Duvoisin reported their findings, which included postmortem examinations of two family members who showed typical Lewy bodies in the substantia nigra.[11]

A total of 400 descendants from a couple who lived in Contursi in the late seventeenth century generated 61 members with Parkinson's, making it the largest known extended family yet encountered and the first that included postmortem examination to confirm the diagnosis.

Duvoisin and Golbe's team collaborated with Dr. Robert Nussbaum, then director of the National Human Genome Research Institute at the National Institutes of Health, to launch the gene-search effort. To locate the Parkinson's-causing gene, they would need sufficient statistical power. That meant comparing the DNA of at least 10 affected individuals to the DNA of unaffected family members. On November 15, 1996, they honed in on a region in the long arm of chromosome 4.[12] Within six months, the specific mutation had been identified: it was in the alpha-synuclein (*SNCA*) gene, which coded for the alpha-synuclein protein.[13] This generated a conundrum, because "normal" alpha-synuclein lives virtually everywhere in the synapses of brain cells, where chemical messengers transfer electronic information from one neuron to the next.

The abnormal alpha-synuclein protein was found to consist of a string of 140 amino acids, with the 53rd amino acid threonine substituted for alanine, abbreviated by geneticists as Ala53Thr, or A53T. The A53T mutation resulted in a change in the shape of alpha-synuclein, forcing it to misfold and clump inside neurons in the form of Lewy bodies, as Maria Grazia Spillantini would demonstrate in 1997.[14] This change in the protein shape disrupted its normal transport and disposition, presumably protein-choking the nerve cells into early death.

Although specific A53T alpha-synuclein mutations have been found in a relatively small percentage of Parkinson's patients, the manner in which alpha synuclein misfolds inside Lewy bodies was found to be identical to that of those patients without mutations. Nussbaum, who recently summarized his involvement in the discovery of the *SNCA* gene, declared: "Regardless of the percentage of inherited cases, finding genes responsible for familial Parkinson's *should be helpful for understanding all forms of the disease*."[15] Therefore, the discovery of alpha-synuclein mutations gave us a centerpiece to the Parkinson puzzle, a veritable Rosetta stone. The "toxicity" of alpha-synuclein has since been at the center of multimillion dollar investments from the National Institutes of Health and the Michael J. Fox Foundation, which calls it "the most important drug target in Parkinson's disease."

The question we will try to answer in Chapter 5 is whether the excessive production of alpha-synuclein, demonstrated to be a cause of familial Parkinson's, also causes the vast majority of cases without mutations.

Braak Hypothesis

In 2003 Dr. Heiko Braak and his colleagues examined the postmortem brains of 41 individuals who had Parkinson's and 69 who did not, using a special staining technique that made the Lewy bodies and Lewy neurites, collectively referred to as the Lewy *pathology*, stand out in tissues both inside and outside of the nervous system.[16]

When Braak and his team surveyed the results of their work, they tried to determine whether there was a pattern (Figure 7). At first glance, the Lewy pathology was observed in ostensibly unrelated regions of the body, including the colon, olfactory bulb, brainstem, and many regions in the brain. Those with no history of Parkinson's during life more often showed Lewy pathology in the lower brainstem and colon. Those with history of Parkinson's showed Lewy pathology in the upper brainstem and several parts of the brain. And then there were those without history of Parkinson's but with more Lewy pathology than would have been anticipated, especially in the colon, olfactory bulb, and lower part of the brainstem. In a world in which Lewy pathology means one thing, this middle-of-the-pack group must have been on the way to developing Parkinson's disease, if they had lived long enough (we shall poke some holes at the "lived long enough" part of this defense in Chapter 6).

According to Braak and colleagues, there were three major conclusions to be drawn from these 110 brains: (1) Lewy pathology appears before Parkinson's can be clinically

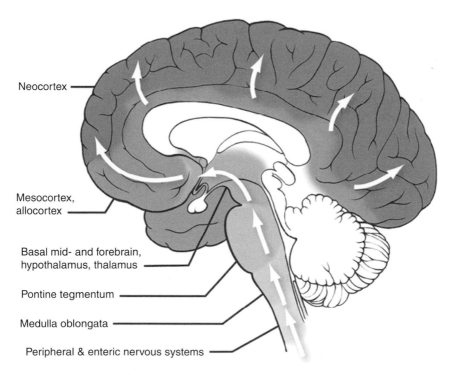

Neocortex

Mesocortex, allocortex

Basal mid- and forebrain, hypothalamus, thalamus

Pontine tegmentum

Medulla oblongata

Peripheral & enteric nervous systems

Figure 7 Progression of pathology related to Parkinson's disease in neurons as per Braak and colleagues. The Lewy pathology in the form of Lewy bodies is shown as "migrating" from the lower parts of the brainstem (medulla oblongata and pontine tegmentum) to the upper part (midbrain), where the dopamine-producing cells of the substantia nigra are (illustration by Marcia Hartsock).

recognized; (2) Parkinson's must begin in the colon and olfactory bulb; and (3) the pathology "spreads" linearly upwards, from a *bottom* in the peripheral nervous system to a *top* in the central nervous system. The peripheral onset was to garner support when alpha-synuclein deposition was reported in biopsy of colon tissue from living patients[17] as well as from people who had not yet developed symptoms of Parkinson's disease.[18]

These conclusions provided a unifying and dynamic view of Parkinson's disease. It also offered support to the epidemiological observation that constipation and loss of smell may be the earliest manifestations of Parkinson's in a large proportion of individuals, at a time when the disease cannot be diagnosed.[3] Although he had no way to determine whether alpha-synuclein could spread from cell to cell in a predictable manner, the data interpreted from autopsy of unrelated individuals with and without Parkinson's implied the *movement* of pathology from one region to an adjacent one.[4] Lewy pathology seem to *progress* in a sequential manner, as if migrating from the peripheral nervous system to the central nervous system, then from the lower brainstem to the upper brainstem, and finally from the upper brainstem to the rest of the brain. The sequence seemed to follow a predestined order, with *Stage 1* marked by Lewy bodies present only in the peripheral nerves of the colon and *Stage 6* when they had already involved the peripheral nerves, the entire brainstem, and every other part of the affected brain.

An important implication of this hypothesis is that alpha-synuclein pathology in the lower brainstem was necessary for the later, predictable appearance of Parkinson's by virtue of the *progression* of such pathology to the upper brainstem. This is the region where substantia nigra neurons produce dopamine. As the pathology "reached" nigral neurons, it was assumed that the immediate effect –dopamine deficiency – would make Parkinson's symptoms overt and diagnosable at the bedside, signaling the "onset" of the disease.

Braak's studies suggesting that the classic pathology of Parkinson's can be demonstrated in the brains of those who do not (but presumably will) have Parkinson's begot an important idea: that there is a long time window before impaired mobility would make the disease apparent on neurological examination. This is the "prodromal" phase of Parkinson's, enshrined as Braak stages 1 and 2. Major research investments have been made to study this prodromal phase and how any of its elements contribute to the expected "phenoconversion," or progression into Braak stage 3, when *prodrome* becomes *disease* because of the appearance of slowness, tremor, and other features used for establishing the clinical diagnosis.[19]

To complement the new Braak-defined world order, we needed explanations for what made the ubiquitous protein alpha-synuclein turn "bad" and how it could actually "migrate" from one cell to another, so that it could impact one part of the nervous system after another. A group of laboratory-based researchers began to converge on a consensus that the crucial time in which the good protein became toxic occurred when it folded into oligomers and fibrils, a journey on which we will concentrate in Chapter 5. Critically, once alpha-synuclein acquires a state of "toxicity," it can also become "infectious." According to cell-based studies, the toxic forms of aggregated protein from one cell entices a "good,"

---

[3] Researchers use the term "prodromal" for the prediagnosis, premotor phase in which constipation and anosmia, among other non-motor symptoms, may occur.

[4] In science, data from cross-sectional studies provide snapshots of events at one time point; time-dependent, cause–effect sequences cannot be inferred from cross-sectional studies. Only prospective studies, following the same cohort of individuals over a long period of time, can establish whether a predicted sequence actually exists.

non-aggregated protein from another to adopt the "bad" conformation via "permissive templating" or "prion-like transmission."[20] These laboratory observations served to further endorse the conclusions of linear progression that Dr. Braak and his team proposed from their influential autopsy study.

The conceptual shift beyond that of a normal protein turning toxic inside a cell, but also becoming "infectious" to neighboring cells, was reminiscent of rare *prion* (*infectious protein*) disorders, such as Creutzfeldt–Jakob disease. As a result, Parkinson's is now often referred to as a *prion-like disorder*.[21,22] Classifying Parkinson's as a *prion-like proteino-pathy* has steered efforts in identifying a biomarker based on the assumed toxic protein forms and designing treatments that halt the propagation of the proteins from one cell to another (More on this in Chapters 7 and 9).

Some snags in the logic of what came to be known as the *Braak Hypothesis* surfaced relatively soon after the publication of the initial 2003 report.[16] For instance, in a series of 79 brains with alpha-synuclein pathology in the upper brainstem, 13 (16%) did not have alpha-synuclein pathology in the lower brainstem.[23] More problematic, many cohorts, including the very one Braak and his team used for their analysis, showed that many individuals die at Braak stages 4 to 6 without any clinical symptoms.[24–26] Bob Burke, whose pioneering findings on alpha-synuclein were to fall out of mainstream because of poor timing (as we shall discover in Chapter 5), used these observations to conclude that there was no relation between Braak stages and the clinical severity of Parkinson's disease.[27]

Although many "exceptions" to the hypothesis were found, with the staging scheme misclassifying upwards of 50% of brains,[28,29] the Braak staging model of progression con-tinues to fuel our conceptual model of Parkinson's disease and guide our therapeutic efforts.

When studies of a family with Parkinson's disease correspond with the presence of a genetic mutation in that family, and the abnormal biology of that mutation is uncovered, it almost always leads to some variation of the headline "a novel causal mechanism and potential target for therapeutic development in Parkinson's disease has been uncovered."

Extreme clinical manifestations (e.g., juvenile-onset Parkinson's) or rare genetic entities (e.g., Parkinson's associated with *GBA* mutations) have been construed as providing pieces to the disease puzzle of Parkinson's disease. This was the spirit of the work that investigators from the Systems Biology Institute in Tokyo developed in 2014.[30] Using sophisticated analytic techniques, they developed a "computationally tractable, comprehensive molecular interaction map" of Parkinson's disease, interlocking molecular pieces as if belonging to a puzzle (Figure 8).

The same spirit has fueled a search for a "complete" view of Parkinson's. In the genetic realm, it has reached its highest expression in genome-wide association studies, or GWAS. Through the power of high numbers afforded by combining large datasets, GWAS seek to identify gene variants, known as single nucleotide polymorphisms, that cluster with a trait of interest.[5] These analyses are unbiased and free of hypothesis because there are no

---

[5] The "trait" of interest in neurological GWAS is the clinical definition; the objective is to find what genetic variants cluster beyond chance, after correcting for the multiple statistical comparisons carried out during the analyses.

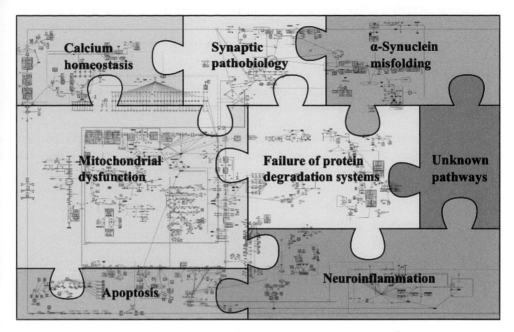

Figure 8 The concept of Parkinson's disease as a puzzle. Analytic methods by a Japanese team created a "map of molecular mechanisms and pathways considered to be the key players in the disease" based on 2,285 elements and 989 reactions supported by 429 articles and 254 entries from publicly available bioinformatic databases. The map shows the range of abnormalities ever described, including synaptic and mitochondrial dysfunction, failure of protein degradation systems, alpha-synuclein misfolding, and neuroinflammation. The depiction into a Parkinson puzzle is a stylistic superimposition on the data by the authors. From Fujita et al., Integrating Pathways of Parkinson's Disease in a Molecular Interaction Map. (distributed under the terms of the Creative Commons Attribution License allowing Open Access, © The Authors, 2014; Fujita, K.A., Ostaszewski, M., Matsuoka, Y. et al. Mol Neurobiol (2014) 49: 88. https://doi.org/10.1007/s12035-013-8489-4)

prespecified genetic variants predicted to be associated with the trait of interest. On the other hand, they are biased from the standpoint of the cohorts from which they draw their data. For instance a GWAS in Parkinson's disease is created from data of cohorts diagnosed as having Parkinson's disease by their doctors.

What may be the largest ever GWAS of Parkinson's disease collected 37,688 cases from 17 databases, evaluating 7.8 million single nucleotide polymorphisms. It found that "90 variants explained 16–36% of the heritable risk of Parkinson's disease depending on prevalence."[31] A separate study of 4,093 patients found two variants with genome-wide statistical significance. One was associated with an earlier onset of postural instability with falls; the other with a lower occurrence of insomnia.[32]

If 90 genetic variants explain about a third of Parkinson's disease, are we missing nearly 200 to make sense of everyone with this disease? And do we need at least 113,000 patients for a GWAS whose output will complete this puzzle? If a pool of 4,000 patients identified two genetic variants clustered around two clinical observations, will the same 2,000-to-1 ratio for patients to genetic variants be needed to find the genetic drivers for the many others?

The finding of MPTP in six drug addicts exposed to synthetic heroin created the fable of Parkinson's disease as the product of environmental toxins against dopamine-producing neurons. The discovery of alpha-synuclein mutation in a large Italian family with severe early-onset parkinsonism and dementia created the fable of Parkinson's disease as a synucleinopathy. The dot-connecting observations on 110 unrelated brains in the Braak laboratory created the fable that Lewy pathology followed a predictable pattern of spread, moving disease-causing alpha-synuclein from the colon to the central nervous system.

These interconnected fables are in constant tension with the reality that no two patients with Parkinson's are alike. Symptoms, response to dopaminergic treatments, complications, and progression vary tremendously from one patient to another. This unifying-diverging tension has made the very definition of neurodegenerative diseases a vexing problem. To that we will turn our attention next.

Commentary – Why Me?

The important thing is not to stop questioning. Curiosity has its own reason for existing.
Albert Einstein

It is a silly question to ask, yet we humans often dig our own graves trying to answer such silly questions. Why me and not someone else? What did I do to deserve this? Why was I "chosen" for this?

In my case, these questions seem even more stark (Figure 9).

I was diagnosed at 29. You know you are an anomaly when you aren't even included in the range of statistical options. It's one thing to be one in a hundred, or one in a thousand; it is quite another to be one in seemingly a hundred-million who will get this disease at such a young age. The question of "why me" then seems very natural to ask.

While there may not be any grand reason why, there must be a reason why some get it and some do not. Surely there must be some sequence of events that can be traced and explain the symptoms I experience. So, I went digging. I learned all that I could about cell biology and neuroscience and genetics and environmental factors, and used that information as tools to mine my medical history looking for clues. This led to a lot of arbitrary connecting of dots as I attributed everything I could remember to the reasons for my disease: hitting my head on a goal post while playing soccer as a kid, migraines I suffered from throughout my childhood, a bad stomach bug I had while travelling in Africa in my early 20s.

I soon saw that this was never going to produce the answer I wanted. Trying to determine the exact combination of genetic, environmental, and aging factors that led to an individual diagnosis is like trying to figure out which leaf is responsible for a forest fire. Anything and everything gets lumped into one's personal teleology.

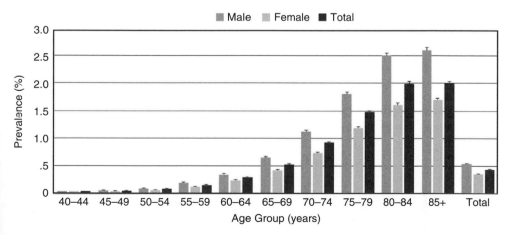

Figure 9 **The prevalence of Parkinson's disease in Canada subdivided by age group.** Although Parkinson's peaks in the 80s in both genders, it occurs at any age. Also note that it is more prevalent in males, a consistent finding across all population studies. Data from July 2017 published by the Public Health Agency of Canada, using Canadian Chronic Disease Surveillance System data files, contributed by provinces and territories and adapted from www.canada.ca/en/public-health/services/publications/diseases-conditions/parkinsonism.html.

But, eventually I came to realize that the important question is not what happened 10 years ago that might have set off this cascade, the important question is – what is happening now inside me that is driving this disease forward. As Alberto will elaborate in the chapters to come, "why me?" is still a very relevant question to ask, though with less focus on the *why* and more on the *me*. Specifically, what biological signatures should we be looking for in each person diagnosed that gives us a clue as to what specifically might be going wrong and how we might be able to intervene.

But to get there, we will first need to more accurately define just what it is we are trying to solve.

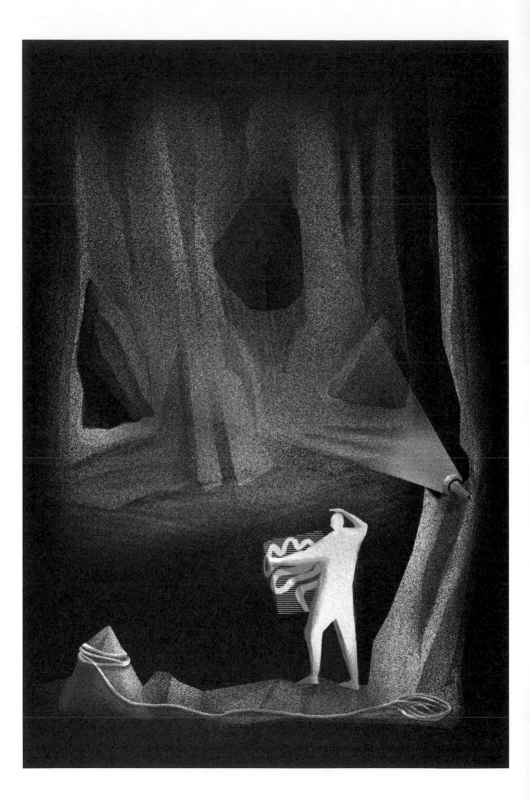

Disease "Redefinition": A Tough Pill to Swallow

Medicine is in the midst of a vast reorganization of fundamental principles. Most of our models of illness are hybrid models; past knowledge is mishmashed with present knowledge. These hybrid models produce the illusion of a systematic understanding of a disease—but the understanding is, in fact, incomplete. Everything seems to work spectacularly, until one planet begins to move backward on the horizon. We have invented many rules to understand normalcy—but we still lack a deeper, more unified understanding of physiology and pathology.

Siddhartha Mukherjee, The Laws of Medicine: Field Notes from an Uncertain Science. *Simon & Schuster, 2015*

The year was 2015. Members of the Movement Disorders Society were abuzz with interest over the publication of a new set of criteria for the diagnosis of Parkinson's disease.[2] Discussions around the world centered on how to put the changes in perspective. How different were the new criteria compared to the one we had relied on for most of the prior two decades? How would it impact research? Could it be useful in sending us down a new path that might finally culminate in disease-modifying therapies?

It was at about the time of this publication that Dr. Emilia Gatto invited me to give a lecture in Buenos Aires titled "Revision of the definition of Parkinson disease" for a Pan-American Movement Disorders Society symposium. She gave me the intellectual freedom to deviate from protocol. Not only was she interested in the similarities and differences between the old and new criteria, but she also wanted my appraisal of the entire enterprise.

As I was preparing the presentation for Emilia's meeting, I came across information from the Parkinson's Progression Markers Initiative (PPMI), an ongoing biomarker-discovery cohort, that was to fundamentally alter the content of my slide deck. The phenotype-biomarker[1] correlations for Year 1 differed from those of Year 2. Further, the Year-1 analysis in the PPMI differed from the Year-1 analysis in the De-Novo Parkinson's (DeNoPa) study, an independent cohort built with a design similar to that of PPMI.

The light bulb went fully off after I read an elegant analysis of the PPMI data by Dr. Tanya Simuni, from Northwestern University in Chicago. The two most commonly accepted Parkinson's phenotypes, the tremor-dominant (TD) and postural instability-gait

---

[1] *Phenotype*, in the context of this book, refers to the set of symptoms, such as tremor and slowness, that make a disease such as Parkinson's apparent to a physician. The diagnosis of Parkinson's disease is based on ascertaining elements of the Parkinson's *phenotype* during the neurological examination. Biomarker-development programs are based on the notion that the phenotype can predict the biology, a fallacy we shall uncover in Chapter 7.

disorder (PIGD), on which all analyses were based, were *unstable;* within a year of enrollment, the TD and PIGD phenotypes shifted by nearly 20% and 40%, respectively, regardless of which treatments the corresponding patients were receiving.

A question then emerged that would change everything for me: How could we be moving toward precision medicine in Parkinson's disease if there are inconsistencies *within* and *between* biomarker cohorts, and fragility in the clinical phenotypes on which the analyses are based? TD and PIGD were the two best-established, widely accepted clinical phenotypes of Parkinson's disease. Were the results on candidate biomarkers inconsistent because the phenotypes themselves were? Were the clinical phenotypes the wrong starting point for the search for biomarkers?

By the time I delivered my presentation in Buenos Aires, I was convinced the field of neurology was trapped in a cognitive dissonance: we had come to accept that Parkinson's was *many* diseases but, also, were ever more confident that a set of revised clinical criteria would serve to uncover the global biological underpinning. The idea of modifying the progression of a single disease we called Parkinson's, branded as the "holy grail" of research, now seemed unfeasible. After discussing these observations with my colleagues Tony Lang and Patrik Brundin, we articulated in a paper that our ongoing biomarker and clinical trial efforts were not preparing our field for true precision medicine.[33] These ideas, along with a proposal to address the dilemma, became the subject of many wine-enhanced discussions with Tony and brainstorming sessions with other members of the Executive Committee of the Parkinson Study Group (PSG), a body on which I was serving at the time. It was at about this time, late 2016, that many of my colleagues came to Cincinnati for a special brainstorming meeting. We were to address the question a philanthropist had asked, "if you had unlimited funding, how would you change the way we study and treat Parkinson's disease?"

The troublesome truth that emerged was that our understanding of Parkinson's disease seemed logical and compelling, but was a biological fiction. This was a tough pill to swallow. Biomarkers were being "discovered" by aligning whatever we found under a microscope with our man-made clinical diagnoses! It is not that we are trying to understand how biology shapes anyone into a form of Parkinson's; rather *we* (doctors) provide the gold standard for who has Parkinson's and who doesn't (*controls*), and then examine what biological signal statistically clusters in Parkinson's that doesn't in controls.

No biomarker candidate "validated" in such fashion could bring about precision therapies. This is the untold story in our search for "the cure." A syndrome, a collection of diseases, can never be cured. Only diseases with specific biological abnormalities can be cured by correcting or attenuating those abnormalities – in those for whom the active abnormality can be measured.

The field of neurodegenerative disorders is among the last in medicine where diagnoses are made using clinical criteria. Other fields – with the best examples coming from oncology – have done the hard work of developing biomarkers independent of clinical insights.

This intellectual state of affairs is wonderfully illustrated by the Duck of Vaucanson and the philosophical school of reductionism (Figures 10 and 11). Reductionism holds that a complex system is nothing but *the sum of its parts.* An example of reductionism in the history of medicine was the so-called *central dogma,* that all life behaviors and phenomena were encoded by the DNA, through messenger RNA (mRNA), and performed by the proteins that make us who we are. We believed that DNA sequence was static throughout

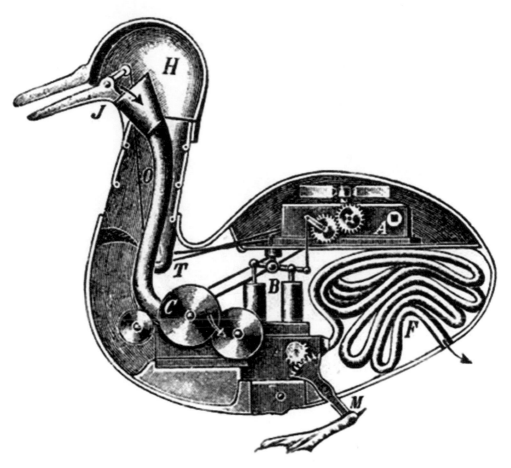

Figure 10 Reductionism model: the Duck of Vaucanson. This engraving of the Canard Digérateur, or "Digesting Duck," illustrated the famous mechanical duck made by Jacques de Vaucanson in the eighteenth century. It supposedly ate grain and excreted droppings in front of an audience unaware the pellets used as stool were not manufactured by the contraption but placed surreptitiously. The "Duck of Vaucanson" served to illustrate Descartes's view (in *De Homine*, 1662) that all animals could be reductively explained as automata. (Copyright in public domain via Wikimedia Commons).

the life of an organism; and that genes were the blueprint for all life.[34] We now know that this reductionist view was an oversimplification: there are many other biological and environmental variables that determine behaviors.

The "central dogma" applied to Parkinson's, Alzheimer's, and most of the diseases of brain aging, is Sir Williams Osler's *clinico-pathologic* model. According to Osler, a disease is defined on the basis of the anatomy and pathology of the principal organ system from which the main symptoms and signs arise.[35] Evidence departing from this model is viewed as the physiological "noise" obscuring the "true signal,"[36] an exception to the rule.

The idea of Parkinson's as one multifaceted disease is reductionist. It represents our belief that almost anything ever described in any form of Parkinson's applies to all of them. This sum-of-all-parts model is as flawed as if we were to say that all swimming birds with webbed feet are ducks, ignoring the fact that these qualities also apply to geese, pelicans,

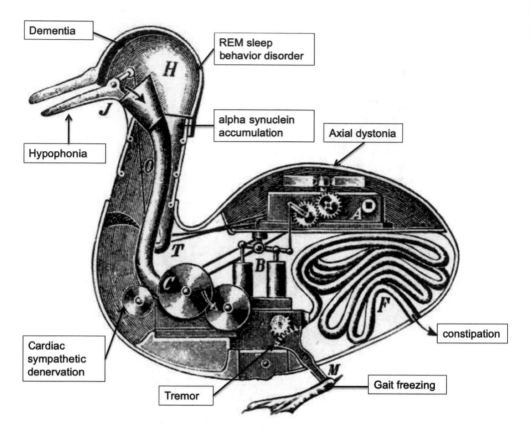

Figure 11 The "Duck of Parkinson." We have reductively attempted to unify the clinical, pathologic, genetic, and molecular heterogeneity of Parkinson's disease into a single "Duck of Parkinson." In this model, each of the contraption's wheels, levers, and pipes is meant to represent a given phenomena of the disease. Only some examples were added to the Canard Digérateur. (Adapted from the "Duck of Vaucanson," Copyright in public domain via Wikimedia Commons.)

albatrosses, puffins, and swans. We should instead advocate for several models, one for each of the Parkinson's expressions, as the many "ducks" and "ponds" that represent this ornithologic family (Figure 12).[37]

The unification of a large range of symptoms into the clinico-pathologic construct of Parkinson's disease has led to many successes in treating some common denominators, such as dopamine deficiency. This neurochemical deficiency can be effectively addressed with dopamine replacement therapies. This is why levodopa, the most effective such treatment, works on virtually everyone with Parkinson's disease, but does not slow down the disease in anyone.[38-40] No intervention that works on common denominators can be expected to slow a disease that results from so many biological disruptions. Each of these disruptions – each duck in its separate pond – must be individually addressed if we are to tackle these diseases.

In neurology we have believed that if we can fully characterize the phenotype (a recognizable collection of symptoms), then we can identify the matching genotype (the genetic causes) and the corresponding biological abnormalities. While this sequence may be helpful in rare disorders with very tight genotype–phenotype correlations, which is not the

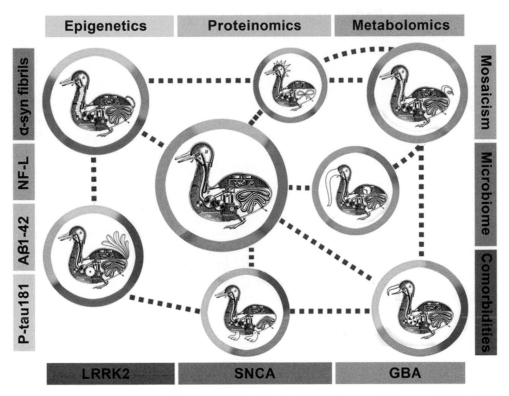

Figure 12 Systems biology: Looks like a duck, walks like a duck, but…there are differences. Modifications of the Duck of Vaucanson illustrate the systems biology model of Parkinson *diseases*. It acknowledges "mechanical" systems within each of these "birds" (representing distinct diseases). Yet it also shares enough external and internal duck-like features to suggest they belong to the same "family," although with a phenotype shaped by the "pond where they swim" (shaded circles surrounding the ducks). Each "pond" includes a combination of genetic, molecular, and environmental traits that combine in systems biology networks. LRRK2: leucine-rich repeat kinase 2 gene; SNCA: alpha-synuclein gene; GBA: glucocerebrosidase gene; P-tau181: tau phosphorylated at threonine 181; α-syn fibrils: oligomeric (presumably "toxic") forms of alpha-synuclein; Aβ1–42: amyloid beta 1–42; NF-L: neurofilament light chain. (Modification of the Canard Digérateur made by Marcia Hartsock; published with Open Access by Espay and Lang[37], and distributed under the terms of the Creative Commons Attribution Non-Commercial License (CC BY-NC 4.0).)

case for most forms of Parkinson's disease, we have yet to try a reverse order of development: to go from genotype to biological abnormality to phenotype (in Chapter 14 we shall discuss how this approach can be enacted in practice).

———

At the end, my "Revision of the definition of Parkinson disease" lecture did not touch upon the diagnostic criteria themselves. The old and new criteria were both inspired by the centrality of impaired mobility as detected by trained eyes. They both operate on the assumption that it is up to expert clinicians to set the "truth" of what is and isn't Parkinson's disease. And they both share a critical omission: the acknowledgment that many biological disruptions yield unique molecular subtypes of Parkinson's which cannot be predicted by their clinical presentation. A truly revised definition of Parkinson's disease, it seems, required a cultural change in neurology.

Commentary – Peddling a Cure

The great enemy of truth is very often not the lie–deliberate, contrived and dishonest–but the myth–persistent, persuasive and unrealistic. Too often we hold fast to the cliches of our forebears. We subject all facts to a prefabricated set of interpretations. We enjoy the comfort of opinion without the discomfort of thought.

John F. Kennedy, Commencement Address at Yale University, June 11, 1962

I have swallowed tablets of bear bile, drank elixirs containing seal penis, had bags of glutathione dripped into my veins, and applied topical creams made from bird saliva. I have experimented with detox regimens, infrared saunas, and transcranial magnetic stimulation; I've gone keto, vegan, and organic; and I have taken an endless assortment of vitamins, minerals, and nutraceuticals. Most had absolutely no benefit, some felt like they did something positive, but on the whole it has been nearly impossible to accurately judge what, if any, effect each had.

The number of symptoms ascribed to Parkinson's disease can seem endless: tremor, rigidity, bradykinesia, dyskinesia, constipation, sleep disorder, loss of speech, impaired posture and balance, dystonia, apathy, depression, impulse control disorder, reduced facial expression, micrographia, low blood pressure, difficulty swallowing, cogwheeling, cramps, numbness, skin problems, problems with executive function, memory impairments, dementia, blurred vision, visual hallucinations, auditory hallucinations, drooling, and a wide assortment of various kinds of pain.

And yet, there are still those that peddle cures purporting to treat the whole of Parkinson's disease. I have lost track of all the claims I have seen made of miracle cures and all the anecdotes of therapies that supposedly performed wonders. In addition to the ones I mentioned above there are many more that I at one time or another considered: bee sting therapy, ice water immersion, conscious walking, electric stimulation mats, high-dose thiamine injections, hypnosis, vagal nerve vibration therapy, antifungal creams and many more.

And then there is the mother of all bogus therapies, stem cells (Figure 13).

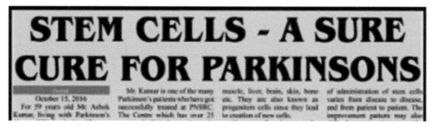

Figure 13 Peddling the cure. Articles like this have become pervasive. Having no evidence to support this and other "cures" has been no deterrent for entrepreneurialism preying on hope.

Here is an email I received from, no joke, The Wu Medical Center in Beijing, China on November 28, 2016:

Dear Benjamin,

> *Based on your condition, our hospital can use two kinds of stem cells to treat your disease:*

> 1. *Neural Stem Cells (NSCs): can be differentiated into functional dopaminergic neuron cells, increase the number of normal neural cells and repair the*

damaged nerves, increase dopaminergic neuron cells' residence to disease, and replace the dead nerve cells.

2. *Mesenchymal Stem Cells (MSCs): are able to improve immunity, endocrine and nutritional functions to facilitate the process of repairing the damaged nerve cells, and increase resistance to disease or injury.*

Our center owns unique stem cell technologies in in-vivo stem cell expressing, controlling, differentiating, and positioning to allow the tissue-reconstruction in an optimized internal environment by using various medications. Our treatment also includes rehabilitation therapies which use biological feedback technology that plays an important role in strengthening and rebuilding neural network.

This treatment needs two weeks, based on our experiences, after the stem cell treatment, you will gain improvement as below:

1. *The muscle power of right arm will be improved, your hands and fingers will be more flexible, so your fingers will do fine movements better and quickly.*
2. *Your lower limbs and joints will be more flexible, your muscle power and tension of lower limbs will be improved, you will walk better and longer, your walking posture will be improved.*
3. *You will be less tremor, clumsy or bradykensia [sic].*

These improvements suggest the beginning of rebuilding process in dopaminergic neuron and initiation of neurons replacement and nerves growth, and the progression of disease has been stopped. In the next 3–6 months after the treatment, your conditions are expected to be further improved with gradual maturity of the stem cells implanted.

At the end of the treatment, Dr. Wu will have a meeting with you to summarize the treatment outcome and tell you what to do in the next 3–6 months for the best treatment effect.

This treatment needs two weeks and the cost of it is USD18, 000 covering patient room (allowing the patient and a caregiver to stay), three times NSCs (Neural Stem Cells) injections and three times MSCs (Mesenchymal Stem Cells) injections, daily medical care, medications, lab examinations, daily rehab training and guided shopping/laundry services. Food and meals are not included.

Our hospital is located in Fengtai, Beijing, China.
If you have any other questions, please let me know.

Best wishes,

I wonder how many charlatans have gotten rich peddling phony treatments for Parkinson's disease? Though it should come as no surprise, desperate people are easily drawn to anyone or anything claiming to relieve what ails them. In his essay, "The Return of the Primitive" (January 29, 1996) Charles Krauthammer fittingly wrote: "In the Middle Ages people took potions for their ailments. In the 19th century they took snake oil. Citizens of today's shiny, technological age are too modern for that. They take antioxidants and extract of cactus instead."

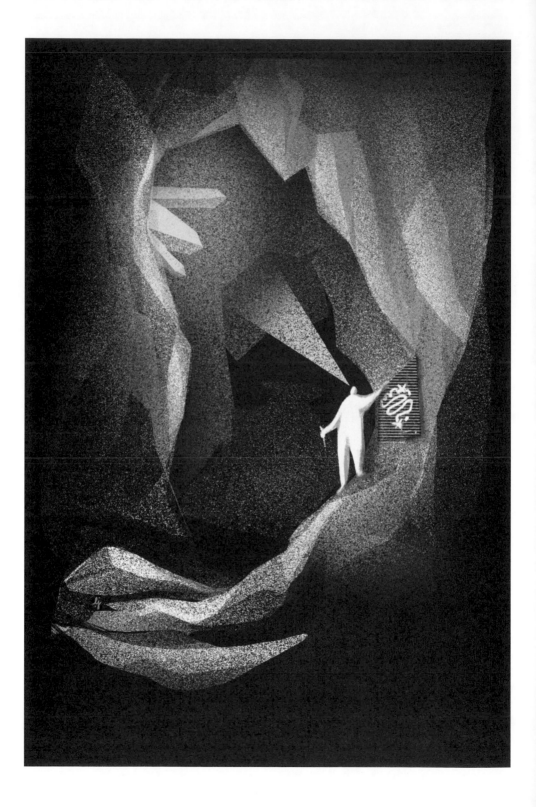

Disease Subtypes: The Promise and the Fallacy

It is more important to know what sort of person has a disease than to know what sort of disease a person has.

Hippocrates

One of the most common questions newly diagnosed patients ask is: "What's in my future?" That question harbors the fear of an ultimately fatal disease, as the "script" associated with Parkinson's is that of a progressive disease that leads to loss of independence, confinement to a wheelchair and, ultimately, an early death.

But there's a dirty little secret. There is no predefined script. The path that any given patient will follow cannot be anticipated with reasonable accuracy.

Here is the most common path: a patient may start with mild and intermittent tremor on one finger, the only abnormality for a year or two. Then he (the majority are men) notices that perhaps typing with the affected hand is slow and his handwriting shrinks. By year three, enough symptoms have accumulated to prompt a consultation with a neurologist. The diagnosis is made at the bedside because this man shows slow movements (*bradykinesia*, a "core" feature) and at least two of the following: tremor, stiffness (rigidity), and an impairment in gait or on posture. If the symptoms do not interfere with activities of daily living, medication typically does not become necessary for another year or two.[1]

This patient is considered to be on the mild end of the spectrum and will be generally expected to progress slowly.

Another pattern may be characterized by a more rapid decline and more disabling symptoms. Within two years, a patient develops shuffling gait, urinary urgency with periods of incontinence, episodes of lightheadedness when standing due to drops in blood pressure, fogginess of mind, difficulty navigating the space around, episodes of visual hallucinations, and short-term memory deficits. Treatments will help, but the expectation is that additional "milestones" will be accrued at a faster rate by that individual and response to therapy will be suboptimal and unsustained.

Patients with mild progression tend to have a relatively good outlook, with better response to therapy and slower time to disability. Those with a rather aggressive early course tend to continue on a malignant path (Figure 14). This observation recognizes the presence of "subtypes." By understanding these, we reason, we can answer the "what's in my future?" question for individual patients.

---

[1] Delaying treatment is no longer recommended, a practice that was common in the 1990s and early 2000s. There are no long-term gains by withholding levodopa, the most important dopaminergic replacement strategy for Parkinson's disease.

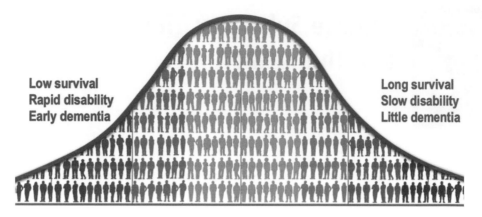

Figure 14 The bell curve of Parkinson's "subtypes." There is no single-disease "script" in Parkinson's. Symptoms and disability range from a malignant course, with death occurring within a decade from onset, to a benign disease, with mild disability and unaffected life span. All of these patients meet criteria for Parkinson's when we define it as a heterogeneous disease. (Illustration by Tonya Hines, Glia Media).

Parkinson's "subtyping" has been a hot intellectual topic since the 1980s. The expectation has been that, if we define and recognize subtypes of identifiable features that seem to predictably appear early in the course of the disease, we may be able to determine not only the rate at which people progress but also the response to treatment and even the individual basis for their illness.

The first *Parkinson's subtypes* were generated from the observation that patients with tremor seemed to progress at a slower rate than patients without. We shall again use the standard abbreviations mentioned in the last chapter, TD for tremor dominant; PIGD for the tremorless subtype. The TD subtype became synonymous with "good" Parkinson's: retrospective analysis of clinical datasets suggested it was associated with slower accrual of milestones and longer survival than the PIGD subtype.[41] However, when applying the subtyping definition criteria on a prospectively followed cohort such as the PPMI introduced before, the classification of these subtypes becomes "unstable"; 20% of the TD subtype switch to the PIGD subtype within one year, while 40% of those in the PIGD subtype migrate in the opposite direction.[42] Regardless of how the data are sliced, there is a tendency for Parkinson's subtypes to change or shift over time.[43]

The era of *big data* brought ostensible refinements to the definition of subtypes. Newer analytic methods of larger, aggregated databases created a growing list of "multidimensional data-driven clusters" of PD subtypes (Table 1). Despite the apparent improvement, however, the proliferation of data-driven PD subtypes has had many problems. These include the startling fact that every subtype ever created has been difficult or impossible to replicate in another cohort or when using a different analytic method.[45]

The most recent entry in the pantheon of data-driven PD subtypes may also be the most intuitive since it matches with three logical levels of severity: "mild-motor predominant," "intermediate," and "diffuse malignant."[46] These mild-moderate-severe subtype definitions were recently applied to a cohort of over 100 autopsy-confirmed Parkinson's disease cases from the Queen Square Brain Bank in London to determine whether these categories, when established within a year from symptom onset, hold in the long term.[47] The longest survival

Table 1 Data-driven Parkinson's disease subtypes

Year created (first author)	Name of Parkinson's Subtypes Created

1999 (Graham)	1. Short duration (mean 5 years):
	  1a. Good motor control without cognitive impairment
	  1b. Good motor control, executive cognitive deficits
	  1c. Older age at onset, poor motor control + complications, mild cognitive impairment
	2. Longer duration (mean 14 years):
	  2a. Poor motor control, no cognitive impairment
	  2b. Poor motor control, moderately severe cognitive impairment

2002 (Gasparoli)	1. Rapid progression 2. Slow progression
2004 (Dujardin)	1. Mild motor impairment, relatively preserved cognition 2. Reduced overall cognitive efficiency, subcortico-frontal syndrome and more severe motor dysfunction
2005 (Lewis)	1. Young onset 2. Non-tremor dominant, cognitive impairment and depression 3. Rapid progression without cognitive impairment 4. Tremor dominant
2006 (Schrag)	1. Young onset 2. Older onset, more rapid progression, less dyskinesias and fluctuations
2008 (Post)	1. Young onset with slow progression 2. Intermediate age onset with anxiety and depression 3. Oldest onset
2009 (Reijnders)	1. Rapid progression 2. Young onset with motor complications 3. Non-tremor dominant and psychopathology 4. Tremor dominant
2011 (Van Rooden)	1. Mild all domains, young 2. Severe motor complications, sleep and depressive 3. symptoms, youngest 4. Medium severity, older 5. Most severe, except mild tremor, prominent motor 6. complications, older
2011 (Liu)	1. Non-tremor dominant 2. Rapid disease progression 3. Young onset 4. Tremor dominant
2017 (Fereshtehnejad)	1. Mild-motor predominant 2. Intermediate 3. Diffuse malignant

Modified and updated from Marras and Lang, "Parkinson's disease subtypes: lost in translation?"[44]

and slowest progression was documented in those in the mild motor-predominant group; the shortest survival and fastest progression in the diffuse malignant group; and the intermediate progression and survival in the intermediate group. The slope of PD progression seemed to be as predictable as suspected.

But do data-driven subtypes match up with the very pathology we consider diagnostic of Parkinson's disease? Is the mild subtype associated with mild pathology and the diffuse malignant subtype with severe pathology? Based on the same study from the Queen Square Brain Bank mentioned above, the answer is a definite *no*.[48] The protein aggregates considered diagnostic for Parkinson's disease (the Lewy bodies) varied in neither severity nor distribution among the Parkinson subtypes (Figure 15). Even when the proteins of Alzheimer's disease (amyloid plaques and tau-filled tangles) are included, the outcome was the same. There was no correlation between any severity-based phenotype and what was found at autopsy.

This observation is not what neurologists learn during training, namely that neurological features reflect the distribution of pathology in the brain. How can we explain this disconnect between the clinical features of Parkinson's and the brain pathology?

Researchers have held on to the notion that the answer lies in a more complete understanding of the pathology itself, in identifying specific conformational shapes of aggregated proteins, particularly their "toxic" forms (oligomers and fibrils). Only then will we

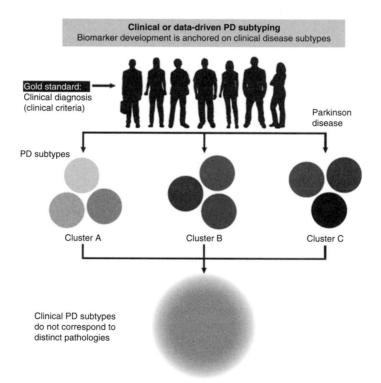

Figure 15 Current Parkinson's disease subtyping strategy. After the clinical diagnosis by a neurologist at the bedside, the "data-driven" subtypes have been created as the "gold standard" against which to analyze what might differ about them. Clusters A–C in this figure correspond to the mild, intermediate, and diffuse malignant subtypes used in the Queen Square Brain Bank study discussed in the text.[47] These subtypes did not differ from each other on any of the pathologic findings at autopsy. Figure from Espay and Marras,[48] reprinted with permission from Springer Nature.

understand how clinical phenotypes are explained and determine the type of biomarkers we need. This rabbit hole of aggregated proteins as the pathology center of the neurodegenerative universe will be the subject of our next chapter.

Commentary – "How Long Do I Have, Doc?"

I wanted a perfect ending. Now I've learned, the hard way, that some poems don't rhyme, and some stories don't have a clear beginning, middle, and end. Life is about not knowing, having to change, taking the moment and making the best of it, without knowing what's going to happen next. Delicious Ambiguity.

Gilda Radner

"What's in my future?" Well, I'm no doctor, but to anyone newly diagnosed, I can tell you exactly what is in your future – uncertainty. No one can accurately tell you how fast you will progress, which symptoms you will get, how long you will be able to work, when you will need a wheelchair, or when this will kill you. And all along the way you will have far more questions than the field is able to answer.

This uncertainty extends to every moment of every day you live with Parkinson's. The number of factors that go into determining how your symptoms will manifest from moment to moment is what makes this disease so difficult to manage. Everything from the amount of sleep you got the night before, to the food you ate throughout the day, to the exact timing of your medication, to your anxiety and stress levels, to how well hydrated you are, and much more all factor into how your symptoms get expressed in a given moment.

As Alberto mentioned above, Parkinson's does not follow a script. There are some patterns and trends in the data that seem to hold in the long term, but with how much confidence can anyone say that any individual falls neatly into any one specific subtype? And what is a patient and their doctor to do with that information?

Almost everything we "know" about this disease comes from studies into groups of people. Those people get plotted as dots on a graph, a line then gets drawn through the middle of the group reflecting the group's average, that average becomes the result of the study, an average that almost none of the dots fall on.

This gets at the importance of what Alberto is proposing. We need to move away from "clinical subtypes" that lump everyone diagnosed with the disease into the same research studies, and towards specific "biological subtypes" associated with biomarkers that we can then develop targeted therapeutic strategies for.

Thankfully, this idea seems to be catching on. In an interview with Dr. Todd Sherer, CEO of the Michael J. Fox Foundation I asked, "What do you believe are the most important unsolved questions in PD research today?" This was his response:

> What I see as most important is trying to get a better biological understanding of the variability in Parkinson's. Some specialists say that when you've met one person with Parkinson's, you've met one person with Parkinson's. But we need to move this beyond phenomenology and into understanding by identifying biological subgroups of the disease and then develop very specific biological targets against that subgroup. Also, why do some people progress more quickly than others? Why do some people get it earlier than others? And then can we turn that understanding into directed therapies? [Jan24, 2018]

I should point out, however, that this is by no means the consensus for how we should move forward. According to Andrew Lees, who from 1985 to 2010 was the most cited investigator in Parkinson's research,[49] "The assumption that understanding molecular mechanisms causing cell death will lead to cures is not justified on the basis of the last 50 years of research."

The field is in flux right now. People are choosing sides, and most researchers are preoccupied with doing whatever they can to drum up interest in what they happen to be working on. It is a turbulent time, and probably will continue to be until someone can put forth incontrovertible proof that something works. But I fear that we won't get there without a critical reappraisal of our fundamental tenets, starting with the very proteins believed to be at the heart of all this dysfunction.

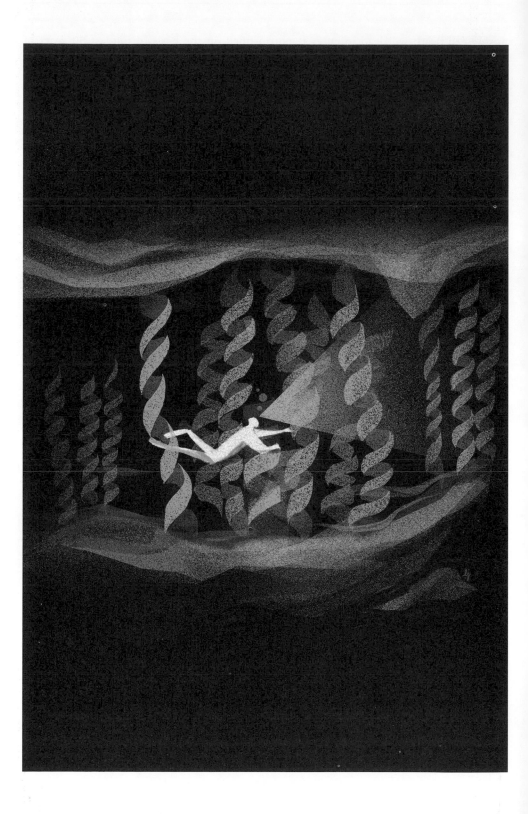

Chapter 5

Protein Paradox

There is nothing more deceptive than an obvious fact.
Arthur Conan Doyle, *The Boscombe Valley Mystery*

In Chapter 4 we reviewed the findings of an important study that demonstrated an ostensible paradox: when we divide patients into subtypes, based on mild, intermediate, and "diffuse malignant" levels of severity, the brain pathology at autopsy does not vary between groups in either severity or distribution. In this chapter, we will examine an even more difficult paradox: the proteins that get identified at autopsy to confirm a diagnosis may have nothing to do with why neurons die.

Let's start with a striking finding from the same autopsy study on clinical subtypes that was overlooked by the authors.[47] Beta-amyloid plaques and tau-filled tangles, which are considered the traditional protein aggregates in the brains of patients with Alzheimer's disease rather than in the brains of patients with Parkinson's disease, were associated with an older age at death. This is to say, patients with Parkinson's disease who had *more* Alzheimer-type pathology in their brains *lived longer*. This makes no sense if the aggregated brain proteins that define neurodegenerative diseases are as bad as we have come to believe. If our disease model is correct, we would expect less pathology among those who live longer and more pathology among those who die sooner.[1]

How did the proteins that most often accumulate in the brain, alpha-synuclein, beta-amyloid, and tau, end up enshrined at the center of our conceptual understanding of *what is wrong* in Parkinson's, Alzheimer's, and other neurodegenerative disorders? How did they become front and center in our attempts to find biomarkers and treatment strategies?

The answer derives in part from the way we study neurological disorders (Figure 16). Because we cannot extract fragments of brain tissue – that is, perform biopsies – in people living with progressive neurological symptoms, we have had to seek clues elsewhere. These clues are obtained by trying to read "smoke signals" (images of the brain or analysis of cerebrospinal fluid, the fluid that bathes the brain, obtained through a spinal tap), by examining changes in distant areas of the body (biopsies of skin or, as recently suggested, even possibly submandibular gland biopsies), or by scavenging the ashes left after the fire (autopsy).

In fact, the diagnoses of Parkinson's and Alzheimer's during life are only at best *probable*. The definitive truth, or "gold standard," has always been defined by the type of protein clumps identified in the brain during autopsy using microscopy techniques. In Alzheimer's, these are amyloid plaques and neurofibrillary tangles. Beta-amyloid protein fragments clump

---

[1] The counter-argument by the defenders of the protein-centric disease model: people who live longer have more time to pile up the bad protein!

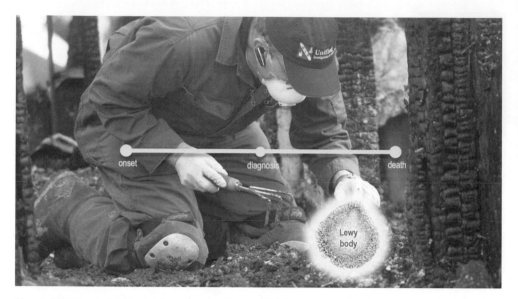

Figure 16 Diagnosis of neurodegenerative diseases. While scavenging for clues in the ashes of a fire finally extinguished, we are attracted by "shiny objects." These provide a "definite" diagnosis and allow us to speculate about the source of the fire, years or decades before it happened. (Illustration by Tonya Hines, Glia Media).

("aggregate") outside neurons into so-called *amyloid plaques*; tau proteins attach to extra phosphate molecules to clump into filaments inside neurons, forming *neurofibrillary tangles*. When enough numbers of plaques and tangles accumulate in certain parts of the brain, the diagnosis of Alzheimer's disease, suspected clinically, becomes *confirmed* on autopsy. This process is similar in Parkinson's. The alpha-synuclein protein clumps into Lewy neurites and Lewy bodies, the gold standard needed to *confirm* the diagnosis of Parkinson's disease on autopsy.

In reviewing the cumulative postmortem studies, we have to entertain a problem that affects the conceptual core of diseases of brain aging: Parkinson's and Alzheimer's do not emerge as distinct as we expect them to be. "Pure" pathology-confirmed Parkinson's without Alzheimer's is rare; most also have enough plaques and tangles to qualify as having Alzheimer's disease.[50] The same problem works in the opposite direction: many patients with clinically suspected and pathology-confirmed Alzheimer's have a load of Lewy pathology sufficient to meet pathologic criteria for Parkinson's. It has been two decades since we came to the remarkable conclusion that "the extent of overlap [of coexistent pathology of Parkinson's and Alzheimer's] is far greater than one would anticipate by chance alone."[51]

The standard explanation for this issue of "*co-pathology*," that is, the presence of more than the "pure" pathology expected, is pretty straightforward – aging increases the chance of developing another neurodegenerative disease. Fair enough. Having Parkinson's is no reason to suspect we cannot also develop Alzheimer's disease. But how frequently could we expect to have both Parkinson's and Alzheimer's and still attribute this misfortune to *aging*? Ten percent? Fifteen? Twenty? (Figure 17)

In 2017, a large study of patients with severe Parkinson's was undertaken to test the so-called one-year rule regarding the onset of dementia.[52] According to that rule, if someone with motor symptoms associated with Parkinson's develops dementia after at least one year,

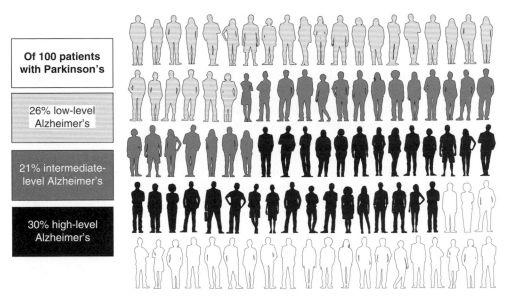

Figure 17 **Parkinson's and Alzheimer's disease co-occurrence.** Of 100 patients with Parkinson's disease confirmed at autopsy, nearly 80% also have Alzheimer's disease pathology. This co-occurrence far exceeds *chance* and likely represents an *association*. These pathologies have therefore more in common with one another than previously recognized, despite their classification as separate entities. (Illustration by Tonya Hines, Glia Media).

the term Parkinson's disease dementia applies. If dementia occurs earlier than that, the agreed-upon term is dementia with Lewy bodies, the most severe end of the Parkinson's spectrum. The one-year rule to define two ostensibly distinct diseases was mostly the product of expert opinion.[53] This study, which gathered brain autopsies from 213 patients with both Parkinson's disease dementia and dementia with Lewy bodies, presented the best evidence that the one-year rule was a fictional creation. Indeed, brain pathology did not substantiate the artificial division of these two disorders within the Parkinson's spectrum.

The most important finding of that study, however, was that it allowed us to look at the issue of "co-pathology." How often did these patients with confirmed aggregation of Lewy bodies explaining their parkinsonism also have enough plaques and tangles to be diagnosed as having had Alzheimer's? The answer: 77%, when combining mild, moderate, and severe levels of pathology.

Compared to other medical illnesses, why would patients with Parkinson's disease be so unlucky as to expect an 8-in-10 chance of having another neurodegenerative disease?

Or could it be that some biological abnormalities, yet to be understood, occurring *before* any protein clumping, brought about protein aggregates in the brain that are currently classified, by virtue of how we have conceptualized our diseases, as belonging to two separate diseases?

George, a 46-year-old man, had been constipated since his twenties. He came to the attention of a neurologist after three years of frequent bouts of urinary urgency, light-headedness after standing, shrinking handwriting, and dragging of his right foot when walking. On examination, he was slow and stiff, and had difficulty copying a pentagon figure and coming up with more than eight words starting with the letter "F" in one minute. His blood pressure was normal when sitting but dropped markedly upon standing. The neurologist concluded that, while atypical, most of these features fell within the broad spectrum of Parkinson's disease. The diagnosis of *probable* Parkinson's disease was made.

The handwriting and foot posturing improved with levodopa, but his lightheadedness worsened. He passed out several times each week. Medications to prop up his blood pressure were added.

Two years later, George began reporting the presence of strangers in his home. His wife, who was often nearby, never saw anyone. Driving became impossible as he could not judge the distance between cars and would get lost easily. Soon he became convinced that his wife was an identical looking imposter. A neuropsychological test confirmed moderate dementia. After a fall, he passed away due to complications from intracranial bleeding while in intensive care. At autopsy, his brain showed widespread Lewy bodies (as well as beta-amyloid plaques, neurofibrillary tangles, and some microvascular disease) confirming the diagnosis of Parkinson's disease dementia.

This case is an example of what neurologists refer to as the *heterogeneity* of Parkinson's disease. Remember, "classic" Parkinson's disease is characterized by the development of an asymmetric hand or foot tremor, along with slowness and stiffness, and a good response to levodopa. The timeline of the inexorable progression is highlighted by motor complications that become difficult to manage after 5 years, cognitive deficits after 10 years, and dementia and orthostatic hypotension after 15. The presence of Lewy bodies on autopsy as the marker of Parkinson's disease has extended the range of manifestations attributable to the same diagnosis. Because of this, although George's clinical course would not fit with the "classic" group, the ascertainment of Lewy pathology in his brain suggests he must have manifested symptoms considered within the broad spectrum of Parkinson's disease.[2]

Scavenging for clues about the nature of a fire from the ashes left behind has consistently led to the conclusion that whatever is found must have been present at the very beginning of the fire, and is the likely cause of it.

The large family with a severe form of Parkinson's from the region of Contursi we introduced in Chapter 2 (their average age at onset was 46 years, the time to death only 9 years from the onset of symptoms), was found to have a specific mutation in their alpha-synuclein gene.[13] The finding was the first demonstration that a genetic mutation could induce Parkinson's. The immediate implication was that alpha-synuclein was central to Lewy bodies and to Parkinson's in general.[14] As subsequent variations in the alpha-synuclein gene were found, including other point mutations and "multiplications" (duplications and triplications of the gene) a "dose" theory emerged, according to which the severity of Parkinson's was dose-dependent, with increasing "levels" of aggregated alpha-synuclein leading to more severe forms of the disease. From these observations, a conclusion was drawn that would dominate the next two decades of Parkinson's research: if alpha-synuclein mutations led to alpha-synuclein accumulation and *familial* Parkinson's disease, and alpha-synuclein also

---

[2] Because of autopsy studies, Lewy bodies are a demonstrated feature of diseases well beyond the broadest definition of Parkinson's disease, which may not even include parkinsonism. Such diseases include Kufor–Rakeb syndrome, Chediak–Higashi syndrome, pure autonomic failure, mitochondrial membrane protein-associated neurodegeneration, PLA2G6-associated neurodegeneration, and Sanfilippo syndrome.

accumulated in non-genetic (also referred to as "sporadic") Parkinson's disease, then alpha-synuclein was the cause for everyone with Parkinson's disease, with or without a mutation, because all of them have alpha-synuclein aggregates accumulating in their brains.[54]

And so Parkinson's came to be known as a *proteinopathy*, a disease *caused by* abnormally aggregated proteins. Other proteinopathies include Alzheimer's, frontotemporal dementia, corticobasal degeneration, multiple systems atrophy, progressive supranuclear palsy, and many other neurodegenerative disorders for which clinico-pathologic criteria have been created. Recognizing protein accumulation as the driving force behind these diseases unleashed a feverish search across many laboratories in the world to conduct experiments aimed at understanding how these proteins clump into insoluble chunks and how they spread throughout the brain. The major belief was that charting the path of these proteins from normal amino acids to abnormal proteins would reveal potentially vulnerable openings to pharmacologic intervention. The Holy Grail became the search-and-destroy mission targeting these proteins. Therein was laid the the promise of curing neurodegenerative diseases.

There is no natural model of Parkinson's disease in the animal kingdom outside of us *Homo sapiens*.[55] To create animal models we use toxins to damage the dopamine-producing cells in the brainstem or genetic manipulation to over-express alpha-synuclein – most often in mice, but also in several other animals. Toxic models have fallen out of favor before because classic Parkinson's does not emerge rapidly after a poisonous insult.[3] Nevertheless, animal models are still widely used in biomedical laboratories around the world largely because of the belief that these models recreate parts of the Parkinson's story.

When alpha-synuclein is artificially over-expressed in animals, the animals become sick, showing slowness in many measurable behaviors. These behaviors are considered sufficiently reminiscent of those seen in humans diagnosed with Parkinson's. Popular methods to increase brain alpha-synuclein in animal models include using attenuated viruses capable of expressing *human* alpha-synuclein, or direct injection of so-called pathogenic (oligomeric) alpha-synuclein species from humans to animals.[56] In animals, the accumulation of foreign proteins also induces the death of neurons, which has supported the connection between protein accumulation and faster cell death, or neurodegeneration. For instance, the fruit fly *Drosophila melanogaster* with over-expressed alpha-synuclein loses its dopamine-producing neurons and its capacity to climb on the walls of a bottle. But when the "longevity agent" spermidine is administered,[4] it averts the neuronal loss and regains its climbing ability.[57] Similar outcomes have been demonstrated in alpha-synuclein-over-expressing mice and rats after the removal of alpha-synuclein with anti-alpha-synuclein antibodies.[58] In short, the cumulative evidence in animals shows that over-expressing alpha-synuclein in animals makes them sick; removing it makes them better.

---

[3] The rapid-onset development of "Parkinson's disease" by George Carrillo, described in Chapter 2, would now be classified as a toxic parkinsonism. He and five others were known to have been exposed to synthetic heroin – yet this finding was held as a clue to the etiology of Parkinson's disease.

[4] Spermidine, whose name comes from "sperm" because it was originally isolated in semen, is a molecule assumed to serve vital roles in the survival of cells, including the facilitation of autophagy (clearance of proteins), reduction of inflammation, enhancement of lipid metabolism, and regulation of cell proliferation and death.

While the artificial introduction of alpha-synuclein, beta-amyloid, and tau proteins into animals creates models of human diseases, what direct evidence do we have from humans that these proteins drive their diseases? We know that mutations in alpha-synuclein and beta-amyloid genes *cause* familial forms of Parkinson's and Alzheimer's in affected individuals with these genetic abnormalities.[4,5] The protein accumulation in these genetic forms of Parkinson's and Alzheimer's must be positioned high up in the cascade of events leading to the death of neurons. But in the absence of these rare mutations, there is no evidence that the presence of aggregated alpha-synuclein alone *causes* all other forms of Parkinson's or the presence of amyloid plaques and tau-filled tangles causes all other forms of Alzheimer's. We suspect that it does given the data from animal models mentioned above and our collective belief that Parkinson's and Alzheimer's each have a common causal root.

There is a major reason we have not gathered direct evidence of the assumed causality between proteins and disease in humans. It would be unethical to conduct a study involving brain biopsies in a large group of healthy individuals, following them over many years to examine the following hypothesis: those in whom alpha synuclein aggregate into Lewy bodies go on to develop Parkinson's, those in whom amyloid aggregate into plaques, and tau into tangles, develop Alzheimer's.

However, indirect evidence can be analyzed in humans using well-established epidemiologic techniques. With a group of 27 colleagues, I conducted a systematic review of all studies carried out to date *on humans* with Parkinson's and Alzheimer's, measuring the aggregated forms of alpha-synuclein, beta-amyloid, and tau proteins. The studies included clinical trials, autopsy studies, and imaging protocols (in this case, of amyloid, the only protein for which a brain imaging technique has been validated and FDA-approved).[4]

We evaluated the extent to which alpha-synuclein, beta-amyloid, and tau aggregation were causal to Parkinson's and Alzheimer's by utilizing an established tool of population studies, the Bradford Hill criteria.[59,60] These are a set of nine criteria developed by Sir Austin Bradford Hill, which, if collectively met, provide epidemiologic evidence of a *causal relationship* between two variables in which one is a cause and the other the observed effect. For our study, satisfying all criteria would mean alpha-synuclein aggregation is a cause of Parkinson's and beta-amyloid and tau aggregation of Alzheimer's.

Three of these criteria are highlighted as examples of the logic behind them:

- "Temporal sequence" necessitates that the variable corresponding to the presumed cause must come before the variable corresponding to the presumed effect.
- "Dose–response" demands evidence for a dose-dependent relationship between the cause and the effect: the more of a cause, the larger the effect (for instance, greater incidence, worse severity, or faster rate of progression).
- "Specificity" requires that proteins associated with one disease are not identifiable in other diseases nor in individuals free of disease. Thus, alpha-synuclein accumulation should be present only in Parkinson's and not in Alzheimer's, other diseases, or normal subjects; beta-amyloid and tau should be present only in Alzheimer's.

We have already suggested that the criterion of specificity cannot be met since co-occurrence or "co-pathology" of Alzheimer's is common in patients with autopsy-confirmed Parkinson's disease and, similarly, "co-pathology" of Parkinson's common in those with

Table 2 Bradford Hill's criteria applied to human studies of alpha-synuclein, beta-amyloid, and tau aggregation in Parkinson's and Alzheimer's diseases.

Criteria	Result in Parkinson's disease	Result in Alzheimer's disease
Strength	**Yes**: Correlated with alpha-synuclein aggregation.	**Yes**: Beta-amyloid and tau aggregation correlated.
Consistency	**Yes**: Consistent correlation between alpha-synuclein with Parkinson's.	**Yes**: Consistent correlation between beta-amyloid/tau aggregates and Alzheimer's.
Temporal sequence	**No**: No studies able to assess in vivo the time interval between alpha-synuclein aggregation and symptom development in Parkinson's.	**Yes**: Beta amyloid/tau aggregation ascertained in vivo before symptom development in Alzheimer's.
Experimental evidence	**No**: Interventions targeted against alpha-synuclein aggregates not yet shown to decrease Parkinson's incidence, severity, or rate of progression.	**No**: Interventions targeted against beta-amyloid/tau aggregates not shown to decrease Alzheimer's incidence, severity, or rate of progression.
Dose–response	**No**: No dose–response curve between alpha-synuclein aggregates concentration and Parkinson's incidence, severity, or rate of progression.	**Yes**: Dose–response curve between beta-amyloid/tau aggregates concentration and Alzheimer's incidence, severity, or rate of progression.
Biological plausibility	**Uncertain**: Evidence for and against alpha-synuclein aggregates leading to molecular pathways associated with Parkinson's.	**Equivocal**: Evidence for and against that beta-amyloid/tau aggregates lead to molecular pathways associated with Alzheimer's.
Analogy	**Circular reasoning**: Parkinson's is pathologically defined by alpha-synuclein aggregates; this criterion is void, given circular reasoning.	**Circular reasoning**: As Alzheimer's is pathologically defined by beta-amyloid/tau aggregates, this criterion is void, given circular reasoning.
Specificity	**No**: If alpha-synuclein aggregates cause Parkinson's, these proteins should not be present in other diseases or healthy controls, yet they are.	**No**: If beta-amyloid/tau aggregates cause Alzheimer's, these proteins should not be present in other diseases or healthy controls, yet they are.
Coherence	**No**: Relationship between alpha-synuclein aggregates and Parkinson's is inconsistent in the available evidence, with contradictions or discrepancies.	**No**: Relationship between beta-amyloid/tau aggregates and Alzheimer's is inconsistent in the available evidence, with contradictions or discrepancies.

For those interested in the set of individual characteristics of supporting and opposing studies for all criteria, please check the supplementary material of the paper "Revisiting Protein Aggregation as Pathogenic in Sporadic Parkinson's and Alzheimer's Diseases."[4]

autopsy-confirmed Alzheimer's disease. What about the other Bradford Hill criteria? For Parkinson's, only two of the criteria supported causality. Five were against and two were inconclusive (evidence split between studies for and against). For Alzheimer's, only four criteria satisfied causality (Table 2).

So, according the Bradford Hill criteria, the available evidence does not support the hypothesis that the accumulation of proteins *causes* Parkinson's or Alzheimer's – even if we continue to use them to define these ostensibly unique diseases and articulate the therapeutic program against them.

———

Around the same time alpha-synuclein took center stage in the world of Parkinson's with the discovery in 1997 of the large family from Contursi, Italy, Dr. Robert Burke and his team from Columbia University were approaching it from a completely different angle. Burke had been focused on axons, the part of the neurons he believed most vulnerable to injury. The axons in which he was most interested were those of the nigrostriatal neurons, arising in the substantia nigra, in the upper brainstem, and responsible for generating the bulk of dopamine and transferring it to the rest of the brain. He wanted to disentangle the mechanisms at play in both the death and survival of these dopamine-producing neurons and how the exposed axons were targeted.

In the early 1990s, Burke had uncovered all signs of *apoptosis*, also known as "programmed cell death," using clumps of chromatin first,[61] and caspase activation later.[5],[62] He and one of his laboratory members, Nikolai Kholodilov, added in 1999 a molecular technique known as "mRNA differential display" to explore the messages that were altered in his models of developmental cell death and axon regeneration. Remarkably, he found that the major protein expressed during regeneration by the substantia nigra was alpha-synuclein.[63] The increased alpha-synuclein mRNA was associated nearly exclusively with surviving neurons and was decreased in dying neurons.[64] He concluded that alpha-synuclein aggregation was "unlikely to play a direct role in apoptotic death in dopamine neurons" and was "more likely to play a role in protection or restoration of neurons which survive."[64] More definitively, he and his team concluded that alpha-synuclein "upregulation" was "a compensatory response in neurons destined to survive."[63]

These data showing alpha-synuclein aggregation acting as a compensatory, protective strategy against mechanisms of cell death were to appear in the midst of a world obsessing over a more ominous role for this protein. His findings in neurotoxic models of Parkinson's disease were at odds with those of the "real world" posed by the Contursi Parkinson's family, in which alpha-synuclein was the central villain well beyond those living in a small Italian town.

Using a very different experimental design in 2001, Burke and his team again concluded "there is no correlation between synuclein expression and apoptotic death" but relegated the role of alpha-synuclein as "likely [representing] a component of a late neuronal maturational response."[65] That same year, he wrote a review titled *Alpha-Synuclein and Parkin: Coming Together of Pieces in Puzzle of Parkinson's Disease*, in which he argued that "Parkinson's disease entered the realm of diseases attributed to toxic protein aggregation joining Alzheimer's disease."[66] He came to embrace the "toxicity" of alpha-synuclein aggregation despite his own research.

---

[5] Chromatin refers to the protein, RNA, and DNA of the chromosomes. Caspase are a specific family of enzymes playing essential roles in programmed cell death.

There is a trace of irony in Burke's change of mind. In the *Pieces in Puzzle* article, he favored the convergence of Parkinson's into a single disease entity using data from the alpha-synuclein-mutated family. He also endorsed the presence of an autosomal recessive form of Parkinson's disease due to deletions in the *PRKN* (parkin) gene, first recognized just a couple of years earlier, in 1998.[67] Remarkably, the brains of individuals with parkin-related parkinsonism, largely of juvenile onset, *lack* alpha-synuclein pathology. The argument of Parkinson's as one proteinopathy puzzle thus had a fatal flaw: it included pieces that did not accumulate protein.

The evidence from the Burke laboratory suggesting alpha-synuclein aggregation is a protective mechanism was to be buried under the long shadow cast by the Contursi Effect, which permeated almost every research endeavor for decades to come. How could alpha-synuclein aggregation be anything but a mechanism of cell death?

In 2004, Bob Burke's team embarked on what was to become their last exploration of alpha-synuclein, and this time they sought a bridge to the body of knowledge the Contursi family had begun to shape. With Drs. Leonidas Stefanis and Bill Dauer, Burke decided to study newborn mice that had normal capacity to over-express alpha-synuclein ("wild-type") and those without such capacity ("null-type"), a novel model in search of a novel result. They examined how neurons from the sympathetic nervous system[6] respond to the deprivation of a natural fertilizer for the brain, nerve growth factor, as a trigger for apoptosis.[68] They found no differences between the "wild" and "null" mice in their susceptibility to the removal of nerve growth factor. The team now concluded that "alpha-synuclein is neither a proapoptotic nor an antiapoptotic mediator in the nervous system."[68]

How can we then explain the previously reported studies, which, for the most part, support an antiapoptotic function for wild-type alpha-synuclein? It is noteworthy that all these studies are based on overexpression of alpha-synuclein, which may lead to nonphysiological levels that have little relevance to its physiological function. In addition, most studies have been performed in cell lines, with a variety of apoptotic stimuli, and thus may not be applicable to the function of alpha-synuclein in the developing postnatal nervous system. Importantly, our study has examined the possible role of alpha-synuclein in apoptotic pathways in catecholaminergic neurons that are lost in Parkinson's disease. Therefore, while overexpressed alpha-synuclein may modulate the response to apoptotic stimuli in select cell lines, this does not appear to occur in the neuronal cell types most relevant to Parkinson's disease.

From Stefanis et al., Lack of alpha-synuclein does not alter apoptosis of neonatal catecholaminergic neurons. *Eur J Neurosci* 2004 Oct;20(7):1969–72.[68]

These investigators could have well written, *we stand corrected, alpha-synuclein must have been a red herring and our finding that it was protective can now be discarded.*

Over-expression of alpha-synuclein was at play in the alpha-synuclein-mutated patients from Contursi, yet the studies of over-expressed alpha-synuclein in the models now had "little relevance." Under the new experimental paradigm used by Stefanis, Dauer, and Burke, the absence of a measurable effect on alpha-synuclein after removing a growth factor was interpreted as the irrelevance of alpha-synuclein. This interpretation assumed that:

---

[6] Sympathetic neurons are part of the autononomic nervous system, which regulates unconscious functions such as heart rate, blood pressure, and sweating. The autonomic system can be affected in Parkinson's disease.

(1) nerve growth factor deprivation was key to understanding the role of alpha-synuclein and (2) the neurons chosen for this experiment were more "relevant" to Parkinson's disease than any of the neurons chosen for experiments before. While these assumptions could have been subject to scrutiny, the conciliatory tone of the conclusions was more in keeping with the times. Bob Burke and his team were no longer in violation of the new reality imposed by the Contursi family. Alpha-synuclein no longer occupied the compensatory, protective pedestal it had been given in earlier experiments.

The reformulated role of alpha-synuclein aggregate as irrelevant ("neither proapoptotic nor antiapoptotic") was to clash with another influential study that permeated neurology in 2004 and cast a shadow that persists to this day: the study that led to the Braak staging. As reviewed in Chapter 3, Heiko Braak and colleagues proposed a staging scheme whereby Parkinson's begins in the peripheral autonomic nervous system of the colon (Braak stage 1), moves into the brainstem (Braak stage 3) and finishes burning the candle in the brain convexity (Braak stage 5).[16] In 2008, in what was to be the last publication by Burke on the topic of alpha-synuclein, "A critical evaluation of the Braak staging scheme for Parkinson's disease,"[27] he wrestled one last time with relinquishing his body of work to the greatest unifying theme of our generation, that of the "caudal-to-rostral" (from the bottom of the nervous system to the top of the brain) spread of alpha-synuclein pathology in Parkinson's disease.

> The concept that lower brainstem synucleinopathy represents "early Parkinson's disease" rests on the supposition that it has a substantial likelihood of progressing within the human lifetime to involve the mesencephalon, and thereby cause the substantia nigra pathology and clinical parkinsonism that have heretofore defined the disease. However, the predictive validity of this concept is doubtful, based on numerous observations made in populations of aged individuals who, despite the absence of neurological signs, have brain synucleinopathy ranging up to Braak stages 4 to 6 at postmortem. Furthermore, there is no relation between Braak stage and the clinical severity of Parkinson's disease. We conclude that the relation between patterns of abnormal synuclein immunostaining in the human brain and the disease entity now recognized as Parkinson's disease remains to be determined.
>
> … At a more basic level, we need a better understanding of the neurobiology of synuclein. Although there is much evidence that overexpression of synuclein can be deleterious to neurons, it is unlikely to be just that simple.
>
> From Burke, Dauer, and Vonsattel. A critical evaluation of the Braak staging scheme for Parkinson's disease. *Ann Neurol* 2008 Nov;64(5):485–91.[27]

While Burke's framing of alpha-synuclein completed the long arch from compensatory to deleterious, from protective to toxic, his final sign of resistance was an eloquent note of caution. He warned of the uncritical acceptance of Parkinson's disease as a "synucleino-pathy," of turning the concept of alpha-synuclein aggregation into dogma for disease causation. He went on to focus on other cellular mechanisms, such as glial-derived and brain-derived neurotrophic factors. A pioneer of alpha-synuclein research, he no longer contributed to the growing body of literature poised to accommodate data on alpha-synuclein to the theory of its toxicity.

Bob Burke died suddenly and prematurely on January 1, 2018. His original findings on alpha-synuclein also underwent an early, untimely death.

While the struggle with alpha-synuclein has been one of connecting disparate pieces to a rickety puzzle, amyloid has wrought an all-out war of attrition. Amyloid is hypothesized to be responsible for Alzheimer's disease. Because amyloid can be measured in spinal fluid and imaged in the brain using several positron emission tomography (PET) techniques,[69] Alzheimer's emerged as the best bet in our struggle with proteinopathies. The levels of tau and amyloid are used to define Alzheimer's disease. Also, because we can also measure the removal of amyloid, we have used it as a biomarker to gauge attempts at curing Alzheimer's.

The most aggressive form of antiamyloid therapies have used humanized monoclonal antibodies that mark for elimination several targets within beta-amyloid, some soluble (dissolvable in water) and presumably "early" on the way to aggregation, and others that are insoluble, and therefore "late."[70] Among the antibodies already tested in clinical trials, solanezumab has targeted soluble forms of beta-amyloid, and gantenerumab and bapineuzumab insoluble forms. All of these antibodies, and even an antiaggregation approach (semagacestat), have failed Phase 3 clinical trials.[71–76] (In Chapter 10 we will add a few extra wrinkles to this story).

The negative conclusion reached by the investigators in these trials is based on the failure of the interventions to show global improvements in the trial participants. But this is only part of the story. The other part is remarkably under-emphasized. In all trials, the experimental interventions were shown to do what they were supposed to do, which in clinical trial parlance is referred to as "target engagement." All anti-amyloid treatments actually removed aggregated amyloid from the brain. From this perspective, these trials were a success. The brain proteins intended for elimination were eliminated.

It just so happened that those in whom amyloid was reduced, worsened.

Just as Alzheimer's researchers have focused on soluble and insoluble forms of aggregated beta-amyloid, Parkinson's researchers have charted a path by which normal alpha-synuclein becomes abnormally aggregated in animal models. The prevailing model holds that alpha-synuclein monomers assemble into oligomers, which in turn give rise to α-synuclein protofibrils, the earliest "disease-causing" abnormalities (Figure 18). After the protofibrils develop, many problems are presumed to follow: dysfunctional neurons, poor connectivity between neurons, and eventually death of the neurons themselves.

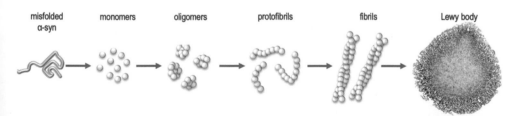

misfolded   monomers   oligomers   protofibrils   fibrils   Lewy body
α-syn

Figure 18 Aggregation of alpha-synuclein. Cell-based studies in animal models have identified these sequential steps in alpha-synuclein misfolding into Lewy bodies. Oligomers and protofibrils are considered the "toxic" species. Lewy bodies, once formed, may not be directly toxic. (Illustration by Tonya Hines, Glia Media).

Electron microscopy studies in animal and cell-based models suggest that the large oligomers and protofibrils of alpha-synuclein impair the function of several parts of the cells, such as the mitochondria and the endoplasmic reticulum. Therefore they have been labeled "toxic." As a result, antibodies against alpha-synuclein oligomers and protofibrils have become a very attractive treatment paradigm,[77] and a number of trials using them have already begun. Recruitment of patients with Parkinson's disease into these clinical trials has been prioritized at many centers.

In 20 years, the war against beta-amyloid has not given us any positive returns on investment. But many still anticipate that the war against alpha-synuclein will.

The lessons from beta (amyloid) have fallen on deaf ears in alpha (synuclein).

The definitions of Parkinson's, Alzheimer's, and virtually all other diseases of brain aging are based on the predominant type of aggregated proteins found in the brains of those patients. In the next chapter, we will review how this model stacks up against alternative models and how a revision of the current model will be necessary if we are to make progress on disease-specific biomarkers and treatments to slow down biologically defined forms of these diseases.

Commentary – Science for Scientists

We look for medicine to be an orderly field of knowledge and procedure. But it is not. It is an imperfect science, an enterprise of constantly changing knowledge, uncertain information, fallible individuals, and at the same time lives on the line. There is science in what we do, yes, but also habit, intuition, and sometimes plain old guessing. The gap between what we know and what we aim for persists. And this gap complicates everything we do.

Atul Gawande, Complications: A Surgeon's Notes on an Imperfect Science, 2002.

First thought upon reading this chapter: "So, not only do I have Parkinson's, but I have an 80% chance of developing Alzheimer's as well. Great, thanks Alberto." Thankfully, as he elucidated above, the evidence may not be quite that foreboding.

But I wonder, how is it that some of the glaring missteps in our understanding of these diseases that Alberto points out could have been overlooked by so many for so long? How could it be that others did not see in the data what he sees?

I am reminded of a quote from my interview with Hilal Lashuel, professor at the EPFL in Switzerland and someone who first made clear to me many of the holes in medical science that I now see: "As researchers, we are lucky that society has blind trust in us; there is no accountability, apart from showing our publications. All scientists have good intentions and have committed to this profession for the right reasons, but we get trapped into this wheel that creates science for scientists rather than science for society."

Scientists often proclaim that they stand on the shoulders of giants. Perhaps that very reverence for their mentors, and the women and men in their textbooks, makes it hard to maintain the skeptical nature that should be the hallmark of their field.

Once upon a time, science was the simple and pure pursuit of curiosity. Someone had a question about the world and they went out and tried to answer it. A couple of centuries went by, and that pursuit became systematized. Now there is a strict order of progression that you must ascend and a code of conduct you must adhere to if you are going to be allowed to try to answer those questions.

One byproduct of this systematization of inquiry is a change in the motivating forces driving humanity's production of knowledge. The goal of most science is no longer to answer questions, help people or advance society. The primary goal of most research today is publication. The entire field uses publishing in one of a selected group of journals as its benchmark for success. Publication history determines who gets funding, who gets to run their own lab, who gets to speak at the big conferences and who earns faculty positions.

These problems were made clear to me by Randy Schekman, founding editor of *eLife* and Nobel laureate:

> *I think the decision-making process is tainted by the profit motive, particularly at Nature and Cell, which are big private businesses. The problem with those two in particular is that, for the most part, the people who make the decisions about what gets reviewed and what gets published are professional editors employed by the publisher to sell magazines. I think this is a conflict of interest. They of course deny this; they say they couldn't possibly predict what is going to be useful or important. But until very recently, largely as a result of public shaming, these people have promoted their journals on the basis of a phony metric called the journal impact factor, which is promulgated by another commercial outfit to help sell magazines. Science [the journal] is a little different because it is a non-profit; they still make*

a lot of money, but it gets put back into the promotion of science, so I am a little more sympathetic to them.

But Cell *and* Nature *are purely for-profit. I'm a capitalist, I believe in free enterprise, and if they were truly making a better product, I would support them, but they are not. They have a business plan that is very effective. People feel trapped by the system and compelled to publish in these journals because it has become part of the culture in biomedical science that if you don't publish in these journals your career will go nowhere. It has become a self-fulfilling prophecy, and they bank on the vanity that scientists have.*   April 26, 2018, tmrwedition.com

To be fair, there is some good that comes out of the way things are. To get published does usually require discovery of something novel, which spurs progress. But one novel discovery then requires years of concessions and edits and re-edits and resubmissions, all to fulfill the whims of reviewers and editorial boards. This process delays new discovery and stifles further progress. While it does ensure that any new claims get sufficiently scrutinized, it is rife with inefficiencies and often depends more on politics and personal bias than science. Along the way it still advances science, but it does so slowly because progress has been rendered a side effect rather than the goal.

Bas Bloem, creator of *ParkinsonNet* and Professor at Radbound University in the Netherlands, put it well when he told me in an interview, "What I see from scientists is that they are very interested in the science, but once their paper has been published, they fly off like a butterfly to the next flower well before the previous flower has bloomed."

At some point early in the career of promising young investigators, they will be pushed or pulled into one of the narrow branches of research that seems, at the moment, most promising. They will then spend their entire careers trying to carve out a name for themselves in that narrow space. And how does one build a name for oneself? Through publication, of course.

But don't get me wrong, science is still the best method we have for answering questions about the world. But the way it is practiced too often stifles innovation and slows progress. For instance, who gets to decide which questions are worth trying to answer? Ideally, something this important would not be up to a few individuals. But that is not the world we live in. Within each domain there are typically a select few who get to decide which questions their field should focus on.

As evidence of protein aggregates accumulating in the brains of people with Parkinson's disease mounted, more and more people found that they could make a career for themselves trying to answer questions we had about these proteins. These questions led to the production of more data, some of which fit with other "key" pieces of evidence until a narrative formed. From there it seems to have snowballed, and any questioning of the original premise got lost along the way.

As Alberto will explain in the next chapter, the story of protein aggregation is a captivating one. There are many brilliant people in the field who came up during the time discoveries surrounding these proteins were made and saw them as plausible hints that something was there. Soon the field found itself made up almost entirely of people asking and answering questions about these proteins. Today, most of the Parkinson's researchers in positions of power got there because of breakthroughs they made in our understanding of these protein aggregates, and their labs continue to receive funding on the premise that their original hypothesis will eventually be proven correct.

It all reminds me of M.C. Escher's *Drawing Hands* (Figure 19). I see a whole industry of people stuck in a narrative loop, constantly feeding the creation that allows them to be.

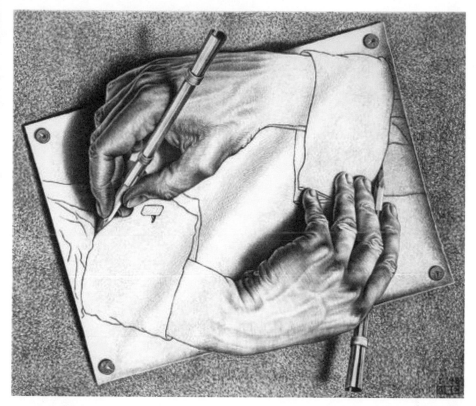

Figure 19 **Drawing Hands**, a lithograph by the Dutch artist Maurits Cornelis Escher (1898–1972), first printed in January 1948. Among many interests, he was fascinated by the contrast between the two-dimensional flatness of a paper sheet and the illusion of three-dimensional volume that can be created with certain shades and perspectives (reprinted under fair use according to United States copyright law).

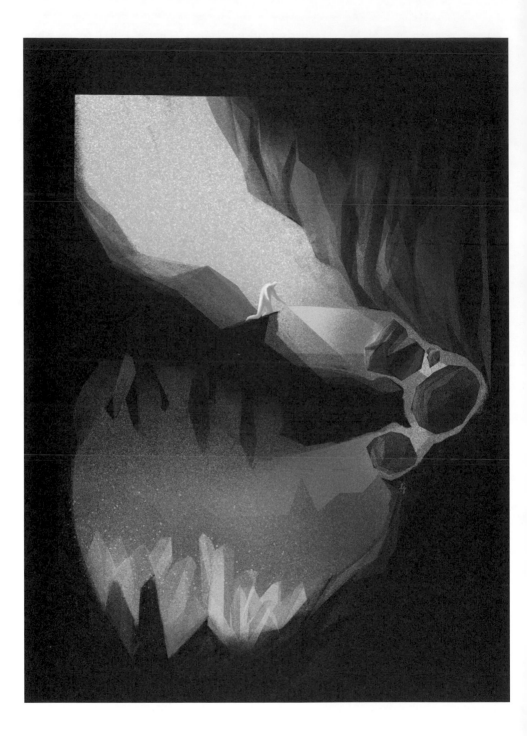

The Fault in Our Models

Chapter

6

Allan Gallup, a retired lawyer and businessman, grew increasingly forgetful in his last few years. Eventually, he could no longer remember how to use a computer or the television [...] After Mr. Gallup died in 2017 at age 87, his brain was sent to Washington University in St. Louis to be examined as part of a national study of the disease.

But it wasn't just Alzheimer's disease, the researchers found. Although Mr. Gallup's brain had all the hallmarks – plaques made of one abnormal protein and tangled strings of another – the tissue also contained clumps of proteins called Lewy bodies, as well as signs of silent strokes. Each of these, too, is a cause of dementia.

Mr. Gallup's brain was typical for an elderly patient with dementia. Although almost all of these patients are given a diagnosis of Alzheimer's disease, nearly every one of them has a mixture of brain abnormalities.

[...]

For researchers trying to find treatments, these so-called mixed pathologies have become a huge scientific problem. Researchers can't tell which of these conditions is the culprit in memory loss in a particular patient, or whether all of them together are to blame.

Gina Kolata, "The Diagnosis Is Alzheimer's. But That's Probably Not the Only Problem," *The New York Times,* April 8, 2019

Aggregated brain proteins are enshrined in a century-old model of disease, the *clinico-pathology* model. The *clinico* part includes the diversity of symptoms and signs that are the expression of many types of abnormalities of brain aging: stooped posture, memory difficulties, problems with urination, depression. The *pathology* part is what we assume brings it all together. If a brain after death is seeded by plaques containing beta-amyloid and neurons filled with tangles of tau, these clinical signs can be safely assumed to belong to one disease: Alzheimer's.

An elderly person aging rapidly with a jerky and progressively useless left arm can look very different from another who cannot recognize his spouse and is getting lost inside his own home. We use the clinical labels corticobasal syndrome for the former and posterior cortical atrophy syndrome for the latter. Yet both, on autopsy, can be shown to have plaques and tangles and be considered, as a result, the same disease, Alzheimer's.

The diseases of brain aging are, as mentioned in the prior chapter, classified by the proteins found at autopsy as *proteinopathies*. Their symptoms and signs converge on the identification of misfolded proteins that accumulate in different regions of the brain. The classic formulation is that Parkinson's brains mainly accumulate alpha-synuclein; Alzheimer's, beta-amyloid and tau; frontotemporal dementia, tau and TDP-43; progressive supranuclear palsy, tau; and so on. Because of the primacy of the clinico-pathologic model for the classification of diseases, a large diversity of symptoms *converge* into a given set of pathologies. Working backward from the pathology, there has been an ever expanding range of phenotypes for each pathology type. That is to say, each proteinopathy is heterogeneous.

We have learned, for instance, that Alzheimer's disease can present with memory loss, language problems, impaired hand dexterity, jerky movements, depression, poor depth perception, disorientation in space, apathy, and personality changes.

Our profession has determined that despite the heterogeneity of presentations, they must all have had the same disease.

But, truly, the same disease? How do we say to a patient who has accrued a mild tremor in one hand over three years, for instance, that because the probable diagnosis is Parkinson's and the likely pathology Lewy bodies, the disease must be the same as someone who experiences falls and memory impairment? We suspect it isn't the same disease but our disease model favors the comfort of convergence while resisting the uncertainties of divergence.

I came of age learning this premise: Parkinson's disease emerges when a combination of environmental exposures and genetic predispositions reaches a given biological threshold, beyond which symptoms appear. In other words, Parkinson's was essentially the misguided and poorly timed alliance of genetic and environmental factors in everyone.

The prevailing model is based on linking genetic and environmental factors into a common final output, the aggregated protein (Figure 20). According to this model, misfolding and subsequent aggregation of a protein such as beta-amyloid or alpha-synuclein is the crucial event that launches a cascade of subsequent biological processes. Each of these processes are fields in and of themselves. A neuroscientist can invest an entire professional

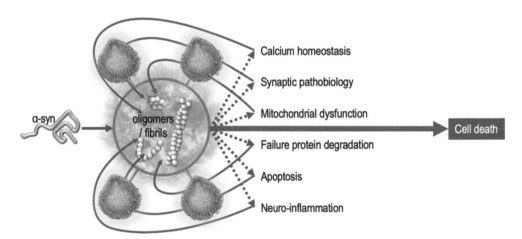

Figure 20 Convergent model: protein aggregation as causative of a single disease. According to this model, "toxic" species of misfolded alpha-synuclein (oligomers and fibrils) are the primary driver of cell death (neurodegeneration). Related biological events are considered secondary to the toxic aggregates, although this model allows for a "second hit" whereby each of these events (e.g., neuroinflammation) can magnify the detrimental effect the aggregated proteins initiated. Shown in large grey circles are the Lewy bodies, which once formed, are generally not deemed toxic. (Illustration by Tonya Hines, Glia Media).

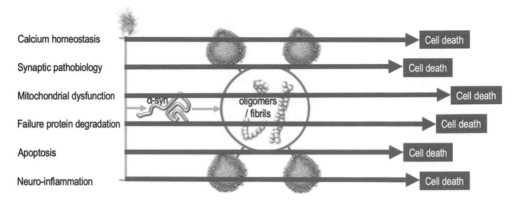

Figure 21 Alternative, divergent model: biological mechanisms as causative of unique diseases; proteins as end-products or protective strategies. Each biological abnormality triggers cell death in unique cellular pathways and timelines. Alpha-synuclein protein aggregates in the course of these biological stressors as either byproducts (inert junk in the background) or compensatory mechanisms (protective strategies) to allow neurons to continue to operate in the face of stress. (Illustration by Tonya Hines, Glia Media).

life in any one of these, along with a like-minded team. For instance, in Parkinson's disease, research careers can be focused on any of the following areas: neuroinflammation, mitochondrial dysfunction, oxidative stress, ubiquitin-proteasome system dysfunction, calcium signaling dysregulation, autophagy dysfunction, synaptic dysfunction, cholesterol metabolism alterations, etc.

The more deeply we have focused on the proteins, that we suspect are capable of initiating all which may be wrong with the brain the more we have lost sight of the possibility that we may be dealing with the end result of many different biological diseases. By nature, we are always drawn toward all-encompassing principles that offer sweeping explanations for the ostensible unruliness of biology.

The appeal of protein aggregation as explaining the heterogeneous universe of Parkinson's, Alzheimer's, and other diseases of brain aging is its synthesizing power. It offers a universal explanation. If only we could understand everything about the proteins that aggregate, we could unlock the mystery of each of the diseases their aggregation has come to define – and lay the path for their cure.

We have evidence that this convergent model holds well in animal models. And so we have insisted that protein aggregation is intrinsically problematic.

But it is also possible that the biological abnormalities we have suspected to arise *after* the aggregation of proteins, may instead be the initiating events (Figure 21). In this scenario, protein aggregates are either end-products or compensatory strategies. Are there any data in humans that can shine a light into alternative roles for these proteins?

If I die unexpectedly and my brain were to be found packed with amyloid plaques and neurofibrillary tangles, the report would conclude: Alberto Espay had preclinical Alzheimer's disease; *had he lived long enough* he would have developed Alzheimer's disease.

It would not be, strictly speaking, incorrect. A substantial proportion of those who harbor Alzheimer's pathology, as measured by amyloid PET scanning, do indeed develop

Alzheimer's disease if followed over a long period of time (this statement will be qualified later). But can we be certain that any future Alzheimer's is *due to* preceding Alzheimer's pathology? Could it be that Alzheimer's pathology would have developed in my brain *in response to* something unknown and yet unmeasurable because it is invisible during a postmortem examination?

There is one powerful window into the relationship between brain proteins and brain aging in humans: the study of the "oldest old," people with longer lifespans than normal who underwent regular neurological examinations prior to death and whose brains have been made available for studies. The "had he lived long enough" argument when interpreting the autopsy findings of a non-demented centenarian with lots of amyloid has no credibility.

It is interesting that the oldest-old literature is burdened with the word "paradoxical." For instance, there is nearly an equal chance of having or not having brain beta-amyloid and tau protein accumulations after age 90 in anyone with cognitive impairment. A person can die over the age of 90 with dementia and have none of these proteins in the brain, or die *without* dementia but have considerable brain pathology.[78] Something similar is true for parkinsonism: 25% of people who live past 90 accrue no slowness, stiffness, or any other parkinsonian features, yet on autopsy have plenty of aggregated alpha-synuclein in their brains.[79] Such loose correlations between the neurological symptoms attributed to Alzheimer's and Parkinson's diseases and the brain proteins that constitute the "gold standard" for their diagnoses put into question the relevance of the clinico-pathologic model of disease.

Among those who lived past 90 with no cognitive impairment or memory problems prior to death, there is more Alzheimer's brain pathology than those with cognition and memory problems.[80,81] This is paradoxical.

Among those with a protective form of apolipoprotein E, *ApoE2*, involved in repairing and protecting neurons and blood vessels in the brain, there is more brain amyloid and tau than in those with *ApoE4*, the "harmful" version of this apolipoprotein.[82] This is paradoxical.

One of the largest oldest-old studies included 127 brains of individuals who lived up to or past 90 and were carefully studied prior to their death.[83] When each of these individuals is classified in a tabular fashion, depending on whether they had dementia or not and in which autopsy "bucket" they fell, very interesting patterns emerge (Table 3). The first, as

Table 3 Data from the second largest oldest-old autopsy study (n = 127).[83]

Autopsy-based classification	No dementia (n = 73)	Dementia (n = 54)
1. Alzheimer's pathology	24	23
2. Non-Alzheimer's pathology	6	19
3. No pathology	43	12

The columns indicate whether patients were classified during life as having dementia or no dementia prior to death; the rows indicate whether patients were classified on autopsy as having Alzheimer's pathology (beta-amyloid plaques and tau-filled tangles), non-Alzheimer's pathology (any of these: "microinfarcts, hippocampal sclerosis, limbic or neo-cortical Lewy bodies, cerebral amyloid angiopathy, white matter disease, subcortical arteriolosclerotic leukoencephalopathy"), or no pathology whatsoever.

mentioned above, is that only half of those who met autopsy criteria for Alzheimer's disease had dementia prior to death. That also means that half of those who had Alzheimer's by autopsy standards had no dementia when alive. This is paradoxical –or it should be by this age if our prevailing clinico-pathologic disease model were true.

The main advantage of this table is that we can use it to ask very simple but meaningful statistical questions of likelihood, referred to as *odds ratios*. The odds ratio (OR) is a statistical representation for the odds that a given *exposure* will lead to a given *outcome*, compared to the odds of the same outcome occurring in the absence of the exposure. The OR is particularly useful when evaluating whether a variable presumed to be a *cause* may be a risk factor for a variable presumed to be an *effect*. A detailed explanation of the rules to interpret OR are shown in the box below.

Rules for Interpreting the Outcome of Odds Ratio (OR) Calculations

- *An OR equal to 1* means the exposure does not affect the odds of the outcome of interest. These variables are essentially co-occurring by chance; the exposure cannot be considered to lead to the presumed outcome.
- *An OR greater than 1* means the exposure is associated with *higher* odds of the outcome of interest. For instance, an OR of 2 means the exposure doubles the odds of the outcome; an OR of 3 means it triples the odds of the outcome, and so forth. An OR greater than 1, therefore, means the exposure can *cause* the outcome.
- *An OR less than 1* means the exposure is associated with *lower* odds of the outcome of interest. For instance, an OR of 0.5 means the exposure cuts the odds of an outcome by half. An OR less than 1, therefore, means the exposure can *protect* against the outcome.

The OR can be easily calculated from the 3 × 2 table above. The first OR is the logical one:

- Compared with people with no pathology, the OR of dementia (the premortem "exposure") leading to Alzheimer's pathology (the postmortem "effect") is 3.5.[1]

This means that there is a three- to fourfold increase in amyloid and tau pathology explaining the dementia that occurs prior to death. This is consistent with our world view: we consider the dementia of Alzheimer's the result of beta-amyloid and tau aggregation in the brain.

Now for the less logical OR calculation:

- Compared with people with no pathology, the OR of dementia leading to non-Alzheimer's pathology (the "effect" as anything other than beta-amyloid and tau aggregation) is 12.4.

According to these data, having dementia is associated to a far greater extent with "non-Alzheimer's" pathology than with Alzheimer's pathology. This is paradoxical given our current model of disease. Is having Alzheimer's pathology in the brain *better* than having any other pathology?

---

[1] As an example of the simplicity of the calculations, the OR = 3.5 of dementia with Alzheimer's pathology was derived from resolving [23 × 43] / [24 × 12], which come from the 3 × 2 table. To calculate an OR we need to use 2 rows simultaneously. For the OR of 3.5, row 1 vs. row 3 were used. For the OR of 12.4, row 2 vs. row 3. Row 3 is always the common comparator.

To resolve that question, we can now calculate the exposure-effect relationship in reverse:

- Compared with non-Alzheimer's pathology, the OR of Alzheimer's pathology (in this case the "exposure") leading to dementia is 0.3.

This is the pinnacle of paradoxes. The data robustly suggest a protective effect of amyloid and tau aggregation. In fact, the *confidence interval* for this OR calculation, a measure to determine if the estimate generated may be unstable, is between 0.1 and 0.9 – solidly in protective territory, never reaching the irrelevance of 1.

The results beg the question: did those super survivors live for as long as they did not *despite* the presence of Alzheimer's pathology but *because* of it?

If proteins that accumulate in the brain are to remain the axis around which diseases are classified and treatment programs designed, then the discrepancy highlighted above needs to be resolved. Enter "cognitive resilience," the latest avenue of research aimed at rationalizing paradoxical results.

The term *cognitive resilience* was coined to denote the phenomenon by which individuals can "resist neuropathologic changes", that is, remain cognitively normal in the face of diagnostic levels of abnormal, presumably toxic proteins, namely tau and beta-amyloid.[84] Since our current disease model relies heavily on these proteins, their presence must indicate that the disease exists – even if symptoms have not occurred. (In a different framework, we also refer to this phenomenon as disease *prodrome*).

The latest and largest over-90 study listed a no-dementia category as *resilient* (Table 4). This cognitively normal group had a similar "intermediate or high level" of Alzheimer's pathology than those with Alzheimer's and non-Alzheimer's dementias. In other words, these individuals met criteria for Alzheimer's based on autopsy, yet they had no cognitive

Table 4 Data from the largest oldest-old study (n = 185)[85]

Autopsy findings (n = 185)	No dementia (n = 49)	Non-Alzheimer's Dementia (n = 40)	Resilient (n = 37)	Alzheimer's dementia (n =59)
Alzheimer's Braak stage	2.7 (2–3)	3.4 (3–4)	3.9 (3–4)	4.6 (4–5)
Lewy pathology	0.1 (0–0)	0.4 (0–0)	0.2 (0–0)	0.4 (0–0)
TDP-43 stage	0.4 (0–1)	0.8 (0–2)	0.3 (0–0)	0.9 (0–2)
Definite CVD	12 (24%)	10 (25%)	3 (8%)	23 (39%)
Limbic ARTAG	1.5 (1–2)	1.4 (0–2)	1.2 (0–2)	1.3 (0–2)
Brainstem ARTAG	0.7 (0–1)	0.6 (0–1)	0.5 (0–1)	0.5 (0–1)
Cortical ARTAG	0.2 (0–0)	0.4 (0–1)	0.1 (0–0)	0.4 (0–1)

The columns indicate the categories classified as dementia or no dementia prior to death; the rows indicate the type of pathology. The Braak stage used for Alzheimer's disease quantifies the tau tangles and beta amyloid from 0 to 6, with a higher number meaning more pathology. The non-Alzheimer's disease pathologies studied include Lewy pathology, TDP-43, CVD (cerebrovascular disease), and ARTAG ("aging-related tau astrogliopathy").

impairment prior to death. They must have been *cognitively resilient*. It could be argued that these individuals were on their way to developing Alzheimer's disease had they lived a few extra years – but they already lived beyond what most of us ever will.

The existence of a group with Alzheimer's pathology but no dementia, whether we call them cognitively resilient or not, has two immediate implications.

The first relates to the *diagnostic value* of autopsy, and is not particularly kind to our current disease model. The over-90 dataset upends the *diagnostic value* of autopsy, which we hold as the truth, or *gold standard,* to confirm the diagnosis of Alzheimer's disease (and all other neurodegenerative disorders).

The diagnostic value of a test can be measured by, among other variables, its sensitivity and specificity. A simple explanation of the interpretation of these two key variables used to determine the diagnostic value of a test is shown in the box.

Rules for Interpreting the Diagnostic Value of a Test

- *Sensitivity of a diagnostic test* quantifies the capacity for that test to be positive if a person actually has the disease; a perfectly sensitive test has a "true positive" rate of 100% so that if the test is negative, the disease is confidently ruled out.
- *Specificity of a diagnostic test* quantifies the capacity for that test to be negative if a person does not have the disease; a perfectly specific test has a "true negative" rate of 100% so that if the test is positive, the disease is ruled in with complete certainty.

Using the oldest-old data, the "intermediate or high level" of Alzheimer's pathology had a sensitivity of 60% and a specificity of 57% for the diagnosis of dementia.[85] With these estimates, we would have to be cautious about assigning diagnostic value to the Alzheimer's pathology measured at autopsy. They reflect some concerns discussed earlier. Based on these data, brain pathology cannot be used to definitively rule in or out a diagnosis of Alzheimer's disease.

The second implication of *resilience* is that it seeks to explain the existence of this paradox in a way that protects the core foundations of our disease model. The alert reader may have noted that the largest dataset just reviewed showed the quantification of several non-Alzheimer's pathologies, including Lewy pathology, TDP-43, cerebro-vascular disease, and ARTAG, or aging-related tau astrogliopathy, recently introduced to describe when tau is found aggregated not in neurons but in astrocytes, another type of brain cell.

Scrolling through Table 4, it becomes apparent that all groups have a little bit of each of these other pathologies, but the resilient group seems to have less additional cerebrovascular disease (CVD) than the other groups (8% vs. 24–39%). The authors also argue that, compared with the Alzheimer's dementia group, the resilient group also had less Lewy pathology, TDP-43, and cortical ARTAG, and conclude that "reductions in non-Alzheimer's pathologies including CVD contribute to cognitive resilience in the oldest-old."[85] Stated otherwise, people can "tolerate" more Alzheimer's pathology without developing dementia because they have to put up with fewer other pathologies thrown their way. They can allocate their resources to "fighting" only one battle rather than many at a time.

Let's make the dissonance explicit. According to these data, *Alzheimer's pathology is neither necessary nor sufficient for dementia to appear.* For dementia to appear, other types of pathology must be present, such as tau tangles and amyloid plaques, because beta-amyloid plaques and tau-filled tangles by themselves do not suffice.

And let's make the research implications also clear. The models we have created for all neurodegenerative diseases dictate that a given set of symptoms can be traced to aggregates of beta-amyloid and tau-filled tangles to define Alzheimer's and to aggregates of alpha-synuclein to define Parkinson's. But the data we have at our disposal is "dirty," not aligning with the 'pure' definitions we have created for Alzheimer's and Parkinson's diseases. About half of those with clinically defined Alzheimer's disease have evidence of Parkinson's pathology at autopsy; conversely, close to 80% of people with Parkinson's have Alzheimer's pathology (as discussed in Chapter 5).

To deal with this problem, instead of reconfiguring the models to which we have adhered for a century in the face of conflicting or "paradoxical" data, we have deployed strategies to further protect them. We are doing so by nurturing two artificial lines of research:

- *"Resilience"*: research efforts to understand why people with so much pathology, which the models implicate as bad, do not develop the disease predicted for them. What factors protect the brain against the "toxicity" of amyloid accumulation? If we can identify the factors that favor resilience, we could harness them to aid efforts in disease modification.
- *"Co-pathology" or "Mixed pathology"*: research efforts seeking to understand why people with a given disease, confirmed to have that disease at autopsy, also have pathology of other diseases. Why are they so unlucky as to have more than one disease? What factors induce the development of other "toxic" proteins and how do these contribute to the expression of their disease? If we can identify these factors, we could measure them to aid efforts to minimize their influence in clinical trials.

The very words *resilience* and *co-pathology* suggest that we should continue to assume the findings from the oldest-old are "paradoxical" and that we should defend the century-old clinico-pathologic model of diseases of brain aging in the face of conflicting data.

In reality, what we are considering as *co-pathology* has been the rule rather than the exception since the beginning. It has been largely forgotten that the original discovery of the human form of alpha-synuclein was as a protein component of the senile plaques of Alzheimer's disease,[86] and that the central, hydrophobic portion of alpha-synuclein is capable of spontaneously forming amyloid fibrils.[87]

Combining the outcome of the analyses of the two large oldest-old studies, it is fair to consider Alzheimer's pathology as representing a *compensatory* strategy. Like most other such strategies, it may eventually be overwhelmed by whatever biological abnormality incited it. Why couldn't the "shiny objects" found in the ashes of a former fire not be the last standing soldiers fighting against the fire? Why should they only be the arsonists?

Would it strike the reader to learn, at this point, that the accumulation of abnormal proteins has never been demonstrated to accelerate the aging of neurons? In the protein-centric world in which diseases of brain aging live, should it not have been already established that the accumulation of misfolded proteins equals cell loss? In fact, the evidence points in the other direction.

- *Evidence from an animal model.* A validated model of Parkinson's, the Gba1$^{D409V/D409V}$ Gaucher mouse model was created to test the potential of therapies against the subtype of Parkinson's disease caused by *GBA* mutations. In that model, the deficiency of the enzyme glucocerebrosidase leads to progressive accumulation with age of a toxic compound, glucosylsphingosine. That in turns prompts the accumulation over time of aggregated alpha-synuclein.[88] However, as the alpha-synuclein aggregates no inflammation or markers of neuronal cell death follow (P. Sardi, personal communication; these findings were not "exciting" to include in his paper).

• *Evidence from humans.* Quantifying the density of Lewy pathology and the density of neurons in the substantia nigra, the dopamine-producing part of the brain, could determine if one correlates with the other. This is exactly what investigators from the Queen Square Brain Bank for Neurological Disorders did. They assessed the Lewy pathology and cell density of 97 patients with Parkinson's disease and observed considerable variation between Lewy pathology and age at death or duration of disease.[89] Neither the distribution nor the density of Lewy pathology was associated with the severity of nigral cell loss.

Here is the major lesson learned from the studies on centenarians, mice, and brain banks: when closely inspected, most brains show *something* they are fighting against. As we approach the "super age" of 90, 100% of us will have tau-filled tangles and 81% beta-amyloid plaques.[85] We would all eventually develop dementia, whatever this means at the extra-ripe age of 115.

The misplaced lesson may be that *true resilience requires the generation of Alzheimer's pathology*. This is likely the case for all diseases of brain aging: the proteins that constitute the autopsy-based confirmation of these diseases are likely either reacting to or protecting the brain from a range of biological disruptions we don't yet recognize, and which surely varies from individual to individual. Aggregated proteins may be universal responses against a wide assortment of injuries, not the therapeutic target for elimination.

———

To our knowledge, there is only one true "natural" animal model of a neurodegenerative disorder. That disorder is chronic traumatic encephalopathy (CTE), considered a *tau proteinopathy*, more economically referred to as a *tauopathy*. CTE is confirmed when the brains of deceased boxers and football players show abundant tau, presumed to have arisen from repetitive head trauma suffered over the course of years.[90] The natural model of CTE is the woodpecker, which habitually bangs its head against the bark of trees.

What makes the woodpecker's brain different from any other birds that do not bang their heads?

It is filled with tau.[91]

The force of each head-banging in woodpeckers is 14 times the force it takes for humans to develop a concussion. And woodpeckers do not wear helmets.

Could it be that tau *is* the helmet that protects woodpeckers' brains from degenerating the way the brains of boxers and football players do? If so, would tau accumulation be a compensatory mechanism in boxers and football players – until such compensation is ultimately overwhelmed by the relentless series of blows and the brain degenerates?

———

The time has come to move from convergent models of brain disease (all defined by some sort of protein accumulation as the central feature) to divergent ones (the protein accumulation is but a common denominator in the pathway of many biological detours). Only by doing so will we be able to account for the enormous variability in the expression of human brain diseases. If each disease arises from unique biological abnormalities, and proteins accumulate across all of them, then it is the distinctive biology, not the common protein buildup, that should define these diseases.

Commentary – Foxes and Hedgehogs

A theory has only the alternative of being right or wrong. A model has a third possibility: it may be right, but irrelevant.

Manfred Eigen

The more things change, the more they stay exactly the same. Here is the opening of a blog post for the *Journal of Parkinson's Disease* by Jon Palfreman, author of one of the most widely acclaimed books on Parkinson's, *Brain Storms*. The blog was written in November 2013, just weeks before my own diagnosis.

> Philosopher Isaiah Berlin argued that great thinkers come in two varieties: foxes and hedgehogs. Foxes dabble, often brilliantly, in many things; hedgehogs discover and develop one big defining idea. Scientific foxes are "splitters," focusing on nature's differences rather than its commonalities. Hedgehogs are "lumpers" who see the big picture. Physics is famous for scientific hedgehogs like Maxwell (who in 1864 unified the previously distinct conceptual domains of electricity and magnetism in his Electromagnetic Theory) and Einstein (who unified space, time and gravity in his over-arching Theory of General Relativity).
>
> Based on what I observed at the recent Third World Parkinson Congress in Montreal [occurring every other year, the 6th WPC took place in Kyoto in June 2019], current Parkinson's research is dominated by splitters. At dozens of presentations, I watched some brilliant scientific foxes argue that everyone's Parkinson's disease is different; that each patient's varied package of symptoms (from traditional complaints like tremor and rigidity to "non-motor" features like sleep disorders, depression, anxiety, hallucinations, and dementia) results from a mind bogglingly complex interaction between genes, environment, lifestyle, age, and luck. As University of Vancouver geneticist Matthew Farrer put it, "there are many paths to Parkinson's."
>
> Does this heterogeneous image of Parkinson's disease simply reflect scientific reality, or does it suggest that the Parkinson's research community lacks hedgehogs of the caliber of Einstein and Maxwell; big thinkers who can develop grand, unifying theories?

Reading that again recently I was struck by how little our discussions about Parkinson's have progressed. The pathophysiology of Parkinson's disease is murky at best. For decades experts have acknowledged that Parkinson's disease has a multicausal heterogeneous etiology that results in a wide spectrum of disorders. Yet, despite all that we have learned of its complexity, and the array of neurochemicals and brain regions and cell types involved, we continue to put forward therapies that target single pathways in groups of patients, acting as if all that heterogeneity is applicable in one way or another to just about everyone.

So, how can we settle this? How can we figure out if we are dealing with one disease or many?

For what it is worth, I hope it is one disease. It would certainly be a much easier problem to solve. We would just need to keep digging through the biology until we find the common thread that unites them.

However, for reasons stated below, I fear that it is a spectrum of disorders. If it is, we need to re-think what we are doing as almost everyone is looking for converging lines of evidence that point to a small number of biological phenomena. This is largely a function of the way medical science works, boiling down a problem to a limited number of dependent and independent variables that we can tweak until we find the right fit.

As best as I can tell, here are the arguments for each side … (looking only at evidence we have from humans)

Arguments for One Disease	Arguments for Many Diseases
Clinical definitions as a single disease have been used for centuries.	Very few people with the same disease share the same set of symptoms.
Most people diagnosed with Parkinson's respond to similar available symptomatic treatments and their progression can be predicted roughly.	There is a large variation in the extent of responses to available treatments and the rate of progression; individual prediction is currently impossible.
Alpha-synuclein aggregates into Lewy bodies are commonly found in the brains of people who were diagnosed with Parkinson's disease.	Similar amounts of the same aggregates have been found in people never diagnosed with Parkinson's disease. There are also groups of people with the disease symptoms but no aggregates.
On postmortem analysis we see roughly the same cell types affected in similar regions of the brain.	There are many different types of cellular dysfunction reported in different forms of Parkinson's disease.
Almost everyone with Parkinson's disease has impairments in the sense of smell.	All clinical trials targeting common impairments to slow disease progression have failed.

While this argument has not been settled, the field acts as if it were one disease. Of the 72 therapies with presumed disease-modifying effects in clinical development, only 8 target a defined subset of those diagnosed.[92] Isn't it past time that at the very least we hedge our bets and start figuring out what might need to be done to tell them apart and tackle each at a time?

Well, to begin, we need evidence. Our best candidates right now for a proof-of-concept of divergence come from our attempts to target patients with genetic variants of the *GBA* and *LRRK2* genes. There are, as of this writing, eight trials in various stages of clinical development targeting these two subtypes. These trials mark a critical moment in the history of neurology as they are among the first attempts to apply principles of precision medicine in neurodegeneration.

To try and get some insight into this I posed the following question to Dario Alessi, who specializes in *LRRK2* mutations in Parkinson's disease: How much variety is there between the various LRRK2 inhibitors, and will some be better suited for certain sub-subtypes of people with *LRRK2* gene mutations?

At the moment, drug companies are being very secretive about the inhibitors they have, so no one knows what the chemical structure of the various inhibitors is. But they will be distinct. Some will be more potent than others, some might penetrate the brain better than others, some might last longer in the body, and each will have different off-target effects that can be quite unpredictable. We will probably end up with seven or eight different clinical trials, and some might work better for certain LRRK2 mutations. Then the work will shift to finding out which patient might be best suited for which inhibitor.[Sep 18, 2018]

So, just how much divergence are we going to have to embrace?

To further complicate the matter, keep in mind that even working with convergent models of disease that target everyone with Parkinson's, we still have trouble recruiting patients for clinical trials. This problem will become exponentially greater once we start subdividing the Parkinson's population. As Anthony E. Lang, head of the movement disorder clinic at the University of Toronto, pointed out in my interview with him, "How do you screen people for one drug or the other when you have a limited number of people who fit the criteria for entry into these trials? This is an ethical concern that our field needs to consider."

The overarching question here is this: how many biological subtypes are there and how many different drugs are we going to need to properly treat all of them?

The path that Alberto is trying to lead us down is by no means the ideal scenario. If what Alberto says is correct, we may need dozens, if not hundreds, of different therapies to cover all the different molecular subtypes of this disease.

I hope he is wrong, but I fear he is right.

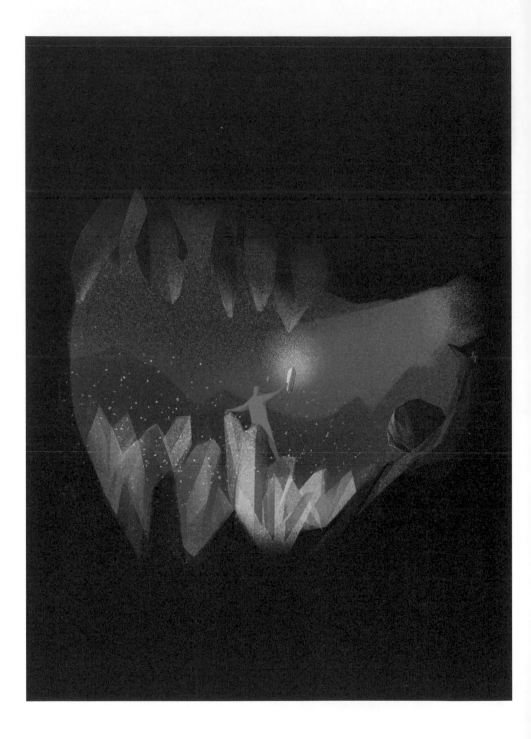

Biomarkers: The Promise and the Fallacy

In theory, there is no difference between theory and practice. But, in practice, there is.
Manfred Eigen

Neurology journals have been flooded with review articles on biomarkers and "precision medicine." Many start with the standard disclaimer that a major challenge for the development of biomarkers is the numerous biological processes responsible for Parkinson's and Alzheimer's diseases. One such disclaimer goes like this: " ... [finding a biomarker or a drug to work on all Parkinson's patients] is wrong because (1) Parkinson's disease is not a single disease, and (2) no two individuals have the same biological makeup."[93] So far so good. However, the very next paragraph starts with: "Now let us summarize the work done to date on validating biomarkers of progression for Parkinson's disease." No further mention is made of *which disease* these efforts pertain to. (Presumably all!) These articles invariably surrendered to the luring power of sophisticated analytic methodologies to overcome the shortcomings mentioned in the disclaimer. The authors believe if the datasets are big enough, the "brute force of statistical power"[94] will come to our rescue to identify molecularly homogeneous subtypes of PD."[95–97]

The Michael J. Fox Foundation illustrated this cognitive dissonance in the Data Challenge issued in 2016 (www.michaeljfox.org/research/data-science.html) to encourage novel analytic approaches on the Parkinson's Progression Markers Initiative (PPMI) dataset, its core investment over the last 10 years. While Challenge 1 asked, "What factors at baseline predict clinical progression in Parkinson's disease?" Challenge 2 asked, "What are the subtypes of Parkinson's disease?" A response to Challenge 2 would require forgetting that there might have been a correct answer to Challenge 1. If there are several subtypes of Parkinson's disease they most likely would not all share the same slope of decline and biomarker of clinical progression.

Unlike other fields of medicine, neurologists remain *originalists,* keen to honor the legacy of our forebears. We strongly believe[1] that Dr. James Parkinson and Dr. Alois Alzheimer, whose centuries-old observations served to define the disorders that bear their names, uncovered not only distinctive clinical patterns but also specific and unifying molecular entities, the complex nature of which we are on the verge of fully elucidating.

The essential premise of biomarker-development cohorts is, as applied to Parkinson's, the following: individuals with the earliest manifestations of what neurologists can define as

---

[1] Sophisticated readers will flinch at the use of "believe" in this context, because science is predicated on evidence, religion on belief. Nevertheless, many international meetings include debates in their programs whereby two presenters defend one side of an argument that is best served, at least for entertainment purposes, by an all-or-none, one-sided belief.

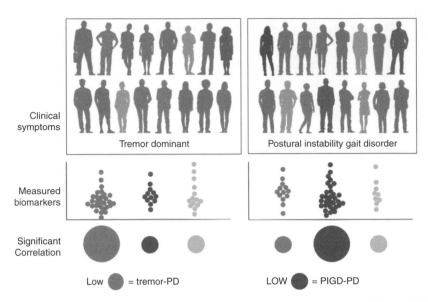

Figure 22 Current model of biomarker development: Clinical diagnosis as gold standard. According to this model, used with minor variations by most biomarker-discovery cohorts, the first step is to form a cohort we can diagnose with clinical criteria such as "Parkinson's disease." We might, as illustrated here, further divide the population into clinical subtypes. Anything we can measure that statistically correlates with one subtype is declared "a biomarker of [disease or subtype]." (Illustration by Tonya Hines, Glia Media).

Parkinson's disease are recruited and further subdivided clinically into however many additional subgroups may be considered. These can include tremor and no-tremor subgroups, or cognitive impairment and no-cognitive-impairment subgroups. Another group of individuals with ostensibly no neurological abnormalities, matched for age, is also recruited as healthy controls. We then obtain blood, urine, spinal fluid, and pictures of the brain to measure as many biological and imaging signals as we can with current technologies. With sufficient collective data accumulated, we proceed to ask the following statistical question: of all biological signals we measured, which clustered significantly more in the group we defined as Parkinson's than in the group defined as controls? The answers become "biomarkers of Parkinson's disease" (Figure 22). Similar analyses can be conducted between clinical subgroups. For instance, if signal X statistically segregates with the tremor group but not with the tremorless one, signal X is a "biomarker of tremor-dominant Parkinson's disease."

But why should our clinical definitions dictate the biological truths? Neil deGrasse Tyson famously quipped that "the universe is under no obligation to make sense to us." The same goes for biology. However, our global biomarker development program is based on the principle that if we organize our patients' entire set of clinical features into discrete categories, or subtypes, as discussed in Chapter 4, biology will follow. We have operated on the concept that the more sophisticated our clinical subtyping becomes, the likelier it is we will find the biological truths that underlie them.

Ongoing biomarker discovery programs include ADNI (Alzheimer's Disease Neuroimaging Initiative) for Alzheimer's disease and PPMI, DeNoPa (De Novo Parkinson), and PDBP (Parkinson's Disease Biomarker Program) for Parkinson's disease.

These programs have been built on cohorts of patients diagnosed by neurologists using criteria validated by other neurologists, such as the International Parkinson and Movement Disorder Society Clinical Diagnostic Criteria for Parkinson's disease published in 2015.[2,98,99] The disease definition may be supported by the inclusion of such convergent biomarkers as a positive brain beta-amyloid scan to "confirm" eligibility for Alzheimer's cohorts or a positive brain dopamine deficiency scan to do so for Parkinson's cohorts.

Now that we appreciate the organizational scheme of the biomarker discovery cohorts, let us highlight some of the output generated by them (Figure 23).

An analysis of the PPMI dataset was made regarding protein-based measures on spinal fluid between 412 patients with Parkinson's disease and 189 healthy controls. The levels of alpha-synuclein, total tau, and phosphorylated tau were statistically lower in the Parkinson's group compared to the control group, whereas beta-amyloid (Aβ1–42) was no different between them.[100] According to the biomarker-discovery logic, alpha-synuclein and tau, total and phosphorylated, could be considered biomarkers of Parkinson's disease if their levels are *lowish* – that is, lower than the average but with an unclear cutoff.

Now let's examine the same analysis in a different cohort, that of the *De Novo Parkinson* (DeNoPa), an European version of the PPMI. In this cohort (123 with Parkinson's; 106 healthy controls) neither total tau nor phosphorylated tau were significantly lower in Parkinson's compared to controls.[101] Only the alpha-synuclein level was *lowish*.[2]

These studies yield substantial overlap for each measured candidate biomarker, making it hard to imagine a future in which each of these candidate biomarkers might be used to

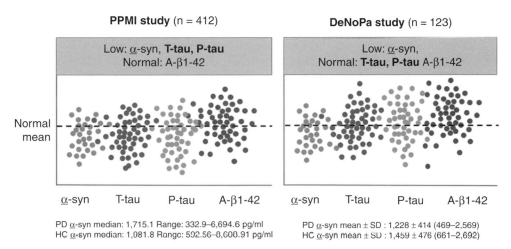

Figure 23 Output of same analysis between two "biomarker discovery" cohorts, PPMI and DeNoPa. Note the large overlap between the measured signals in each cohort. The scattergram is a visual representation of the average data of patients compared to the mean from healthy controls. The data are summarized numerically at the bottom as *median* for the PPMI study or *mean* for the DeNoPA study. α-syn: alpha-synuclein, T-tau: total tau; P-tau: phosphorylated tau; Aβ1–42: beta-amyloid (amino acids 1–42). (Illustration by Tonya Hines, Glia Media).

---

[2] In the same study, spinal fluid alpha-synuclein did not change over a two-year period, suggesting it would not be useful for monitoring disease progression.

translate into improved understanding of an individual patient. Even more critically, the results from one cohort do not match with those of the other. If we are uncovering biological truths, however cluttered they may seem, shouldn't at least the overall direction of the changes be the same in both studies?

A major conclusion is that there are inconsistencies between biomarker-discovery cohorts.

Could it be that the problem is the gold standard on which the analysis are based, the very definition of disease and disease subtypes?

As alluded to in prior chapters, we clinicians subdivide Parkinson's disease according to predominant symptoms, or, as we call them, phenotypes. Our biomarker-discovery cohorts have been assembled around the same concept. The PPMI gathered data to extract what we refer to as tremor-dominant and tremorless (or "postural instability-gait disorder") phenotypes of Parkinson's disease. It also does the same for a range of "non-motor" phenotypes, such as mild cognitive impairment and dementia.[102] We do this because there seems to be a predefined order to each. Characterizing a patient as belonging to a given phenotype might tell us what could happen over time. For instance, epidemiologic studies have shown that the tremorless phenotype is associated with greater likelihood of evolving into cognitive impairment and dementia phenotypes.[103]

Interesting paradoxes emerge when these clinical phenotypes are extracted from the PPMI dataset and analyzed for the same candidate biomarker mentioned above. At baseline, the tremorless phenotype is shown to statistically correlate with low alpha-synuclein in spinal fluid and, consistent with the epidemiologic data, with worse cognitive performance.[100] However, if we examine which measured candidate biomarker might predict those with normal cognition at baseline who go on to develop cognitive impairment by the second year (the number for this analysis is 286 patients) it is no longer lowish alpha-synuclein but lowish beta-amyloid compared to healthy controls.[3],[104]

Here is another conclusion: there are inconsistencies even *within* biomarker-discovery cohorts.

The conflicting and overlapping data from these cohorts have been explained as reflecting the "disease heterogeneity" of Parkinson's. Here is how the status of biomarkers for Parkinson's disease, mostly focused on alpha-synuclein, were recently summarized, nearly verbatim:[105]

- Spinal fluid total alpha-synuclein is lower in patients with Parkinson's disease compared with healthy controls. The risk of blood contamination is high. Diagnostic accuracy is low so this biomarker alone should not be considered useful in the diagnosis of Parkinson's disease.
- Spinal fluid oligomeric [pre-Lewy bodies] alpha-synuclein, and phosphorylated alpha-synuclein are higher in patients with Parkinson's disease compared with healthy and neurological controls. However, further studies are required to support their potential diagnostic value and to overcome analytical issues.

---

[3] As with other putative biomarkers, the values for beta-amyloid (Aβ1–42) between Parkinson's patients and controls overlap greatly. The averages expressed as means between groups are 343.8 pg/mL for patients and 380.4 pg/mL for controls, which are statistically different but hardly useful to identify how one might interpret a given value for any individual patient. Also, it is unlikely that the magnitude of separation between the groups represents important biological differences to each.

- Spinal fluid pro-aggregating forms of alpha-synuclein have shown promising preliminary results as diagnostic markers in Parkinson's disease. Larger studies are required and analytical issues (i.e., reproducibility and assay time) have to be addressed.
- Classic Alzheimer's disease biomarkers alone are not helpful in the diagnostic process for Parkinson's disease, but can improve its prognostic assessment: cerebrospinal fluid levels of $A\beta42$ [beta-amyloid] marking future cognitive decline; total and phosphorylated tau potentially marking progression of motor disability.
- Spinal fluid and blood neurofilament light chain can be useful to discriminate Parkinson's disease from progressive supranuclear palsy, multiple system atrophy, and corticobasal syndrome in cases with confounding clinical presentations.
- A combination of multiple spinal fluid (and probably blood) biomarkers reflecting different pathogenic mechanisms taking place during Parkinson's disease might enable earlier diagnosis and more accurate prognostic assessment in Parkinson's disease.

Stated differently, we know what Parkinson's is, but don't know if we can yet use any test to confirm it. While we consider it a synucleinopathy, measures of alpha-synuclein are not yet adequate for it. There are promising leads but more studies will be needed and likely more than one biomarker will be required to account for Parkinson's heterogeneity.

As sensible as it seems, the "more than one biomarker" forecast is also an acknowledgement that we are trying to fit biological measures to ensure Parkinson's remains the same entity biologically as we recognize it clinically.

Nevertheless, let us review the status of *combined biomarkers* to discriminate Parkinson's disease from healthy controls. The list is complex but the reader can quickly skim through without stopping on details. The idea is to make a major point immediately after:

- *Combined biomarkers with prognostic value*: Phosphorylated tau to total tau ratio and phosphorylated tau to to $A\beta42$ ratio correlates with the rate of change in the motor scale.[106]
- *Combined biomarkers with diagnostic value*: Beta-amyloid ($A\beta42$) to total tau ratio discriminates Parkinson's disease from controls with an Area Under the ROC Curve or AUC[4] of 0.71 and a sensitivity of 82% and specificity of 56%.[107]
- *Also assessing diagnostic value*: Glucocerebrosidase with beta-hexosaminidase, cathepsin D, total alpha-synuclein, and beta-amyloid when together discriminate Parkinson's disease from control with an AUC of 0.83, a sensitivity of 84% and a specificity of 75%.[108]
- *Combined biomarkers for diagnostic and prognostic value*: Oligomeric alpha-synuclein to total alpha-synuclein ratio discriminates Parkinson's disease from control with an AUC of 0.82, sensitivity of 68%, and specificity of 85%.[109] A decrease in spinal fluid oligomeric alpha-synuclein and total alpha-synuclein correlate with motor worsening in patients with the tremorless phenotype.[109]

And here is a glimpse of where we are in terms of the diagnostic value of *combined biomarkers* in discriminating Parkinson's from diseases that may look like it but for which we have different criteria:

---

[4] AUC or Area Under the ROC Curve is a measure of how well a parameter can distinguish between two diagnostic groups (diseased/normal). An AUC of 0.70–0.80 is considered "fair"; 0.81–0.90, "good" and 0.91–1, "excellent." Sensitivity and specificity were defined in Chapter 6.

- Total tau to beta-amyloid (Aβ42) ratio discriminates Parkinson's disease from multiple system atrophy with an AUC of 0.82, a sensitivity of 71%, and a specificity of 93%.[110]
- Neurofilament light chain to beta-amyloid ratio discriminates Parkinson's disease from progressive supranuclear palsy with an AUC of 0.82, a sensitivity of 100%, and a specificity of 68%.[111]
- FABP3 (heart-type fatty acid binding protein 3) with total tau and total alpha-synuclein discriminates Parkinson's disease from dementia with Lewy bodies with an AUC of 0.92, a sensitivity of 80%, and a specificity 95%.[112]

Collectively, the output of these research efforts are *fitting data to purpose*. The purpose is to approximate or match (and eventually presumably replace) a doctor's unquestioned dichotomization powers to put people into Yes-Parkinson's and No-Parkinson's groups. We are not *fitting purpose to the data* because we are not prepared to relinquish the absolute sorting authority we self-assigned. If we were to let the data define the purpose, the output may not validate our neat dichotomous world of disease/no disease but, rather, yield a range of molecularly separate diseases.

Because of this implicit *fitting data to purpose*, investigators used ratios (one measure in relation to another) or combinations of up to four biological measures to bring the critical AUC, a measure of diagnostic value, past the threshold of 0.80 (an ideal test would have an AUC = 1). Notice in the list above that most combinations examined ended up with suboptimal diagnostic and prognostic yields. None met criteria of "excellent" in discriminating Parkinson's from healthy controls. Only some may help separate Parkinson's from more aggressive parkinsonisms, such as progressive supranuclear disease, but the clinical criteria applied for other parkinsonisms, defined a priori, is vastly different. All of this is problematic with *the purpose*.

And we are not bringing back into this discussion the problem of reproducibility, the inconsistencies within and between cohorts mentioned earlier.

These results have not yet forced a reconsideration of the model in which the clinical phenotypes, determined by doctors, act as the gold standards against which the value of candidate biomarkers for diagnosis or prognosis is quantified.

To avoid inflicting the burden of revisiting the assumptions on which the cohorts were designed, and turn the ship around, the results have instead fueled the interest in connecting all cohorts to provide what we suspect is missing: statistical power. These cohorts are individually relatively small, but together they could be a "super cohort." Bigger must be better. The solution lies in harnessing the "brute force" of numbers. Toward this end, it has been proposed to standardize the collection and storage of biological specimens from participants across every ongoing cohort in order to use some (e.g., PPMI) for "discovery" and others (e.g., DeNoPa) for "replication of promising biomarkers."[113]

Just like "big data" does not necessarily mean good data, the aggregation of biomarker-discovery cohorts will not overcome their fundamental problem. They were assembled on the basis of an agreed-upon truth, namely the contours of disease we came to embrace as biological because of the clinical descriptions an astute doctor made in 1817.

How this approach contrasts with that of other fields will be highlighted in the next chapter.

Commentary – Diabetes Envy

We demand rigidly defined areas of doubt and uncertainty!
Douglas Adams, The Hitchhiker's Guide to the Galaxy

Sara Riggare, a doctoral student at Karolinska Institutet who also lives with Parkinson's, remarked in my interview with her, "Sometimes I have diabetes envy in that they have clear measures for their current state, their blood-glucose levels, as well as the HBA1c test as a measure of their long-term progression. Of course, having type 1 diabetes isn't easy either, but they have clear measures that they can use to optimize things."

Indeed, discovering such an elusive marker would completely change how we study and treat Parkinson's. At the moment the best test we have to monitor progression is a motor test performed by neurologists called the Unified Parkinson's Disease Rating Scale (or UPDRS), which Michael J. Fox astutely described in a talk of his I attended in the fall of 2017 as an "elaborate drunk test." Touch your fingers here, walk up and down there, tap your toes here. For all the advancements we have made we still rely on some pretty crude techniques to determine if what a person has is even what can be called Parkinson's disease.

The largest and most well-funded attempt to find biomarkers is the aforementioned PPMI, developed by the Michael J. Fox Foundation (MJFF) in partnership with many pharmaceutical companies. The MJFF has been a driving force in Parkinson's research ever since its inception nearly 20 years ago. Not only has it raised to date over $800 million for Parkinson's disease research, but it has also helped catapult Parkinson's disease into the international spotlight and given hope to millions struggling with this disease.

However, the organization is approaching a rather ominous anniversary. In a quote from Jon Palfreman's book *Brain Storms*, Michael J. Fox says to Deborah Brooks (co-founder of the MJFF), "The last thing I want is for you and I to find ourselves discussing our twentieth annual fundraiser. In fact, if that day ever comes you're fired."[114] The foundation will turn 20 on October 31st, 2020.

I asked Todd Sherer, CEO of the MJFF, "Is the reason why we haven't solved this yet because this disease and the brain are more complex than we anticipated, or is it because we are not as smart and/or collaborative as we need to be to solve this?" To which he said:

> I think it is a combination. The first thing that is very clear is that not only is the brain more complex than we anticipated, but Parkinson's disease is also more complex than we thought. I started in PD research about 20 years ago, and the reason I chose Parkinson's is that I was very interested in doing disease-relevant research in neuroscience. When I looked at different diseases, it seemed like we knew the most about Parkinson's. At the time it was believed that all the symptoms of PD were due to the loss of a very small percentage of dopamine cells in one region of the brain. I thought, that's not going to be that hard. If we can just keep 10–20% of those cells from degenerating we'll cure Parkinson's. We now know there is much much more to this disease than that and the more we learn about this disease the more we realize that we are not as smart as we thought we were.
>
> But how the research is being conducted is also key. One of the roles MJFF has played since starting is to really incentivize collaboration and bring the industry and academic communities together to work closely in problem solving. We are also doing this by developing studies like the PPMI study, which should have been done 20 or 30 years ago, to establish a better baseline understanding of the disease.[Jan 24, 2018]

For two years I was a participant in the PPMI study. The study is one of the largest and most ambitious in the history of neurology. Thousands of study participants, dozens of centers, and hundreds of doctors and nurses and scientists and administrators, all working towards finding a biological signal that can unambiguously tell us something meaningful about an individual's Parkinson's disease.

For me, it was, for the most part, a pleasant experience. I was treated to regular paid trips to New Haven, Connecticut with nice big Lincoln town cars waiting to pick me up at the airport. But there was one distinctly unpleasant experience from one of my visits that I noted in a journal …

> *November 30th, 2016 – New Haven, Connecticut: Spent the morning in a doctor's office lying on my side with my knees tucked into my chest while behind me a neurologist was inserting a catheter into my spine. For forty minutes he dug around in my back extracting cerebral spinal fluid. Almost every time he reinserted that little tube it would trip a nerve that sent a jolt of pressure and electricity into one of my butt cheeks or all the way down to my feet. The discomfort kicked my tremors up into fifth gear and caused me to break out into a sweat as a kind southern nurse practitioner tried as best she could to distract me from what was happening. As I lay there, while transparent goo that my body made to protect and nourish my brain was slowly being sucked from my spine I started questioning why I had volunteered for this.*

As you can see, such studies can be rather onerous for those involved, making it all the more imperative that they are designed properly. In this case that means designed in such a way to give us the best chance of finding biomarkers for these diseases.

This year I dropped out of the PPMI study. For the reasons Alberto stated earlier in this chapter, I no longer believe the program can deliver on the promise of finding relevant biomarkers, at least not as currently constructed. To do this right we need to blind ourselves not only to what to look for, but to the diseases as well. Biology does not have boundaries between what we call Parkinson's or Alzheimer's or any other degenerative brain condition. Each name we have given to these conditions represents a spectrum that bleeds into one another. In fact, the same experts that helped give us the definitions we use frequently misdiagnose them. Yet we continue to lump people together into categories that were made decades before we had the tools and insights needed to accurately define them.

For all we know, people with different clinical diagnoses might share similar underlying biological abnormalities. For example, two people could have the same viral infection that leads to chronic inflammation but due to all the differences in their physiology one could go on to get a form of dementia, the other a form of Parkinson's. Or, as was pointed out to me by clinician-scientist Prof. Alice Chen-Plotkin of the University of Pennsylvania, expansion of the gene *C9orf72* can manifest as ALS (amyotrophic lateral sclerosis) or frontotemporal dementia, in the same family.

Technology to the rescue?

Society has developed an insatiable thirst to turn everything into data. And for good reason, big data analytics has revolutionized everything from radiology to basketball. The overwhelming success has led many to believe that if we just gather enough information and apply clever enough algorithms we can come up with more effective solutions to just about any problem we face. In Parkinson's this has resulted in fingernail sensors, eye trackers, full body 3D motion sensors, and much more.

But can something as subjective as Parkinson's disease be turned into meaningful data? Given how incredibly heterogeneous and multifaceted the disease is, can any objective measure capture enough of the experience to inform therapeutic decisions and improve outcomes? Or will we just end up with piles of data but no real-world benefits for patients?

At the end of 2018 the *Journal of Parkinson* released a series of articles from many of the world leaders in PD predicting what the next 20 years of Parkinson's research will look like. Several touched on the emerging role of tech in PD, but the one that stood out to me was a paper from Prof. Anthony E. Lang and Prof. Alberto Espay. (Yes, *that* Alberto Espay!) Among their many thought-provoking predictions, the authors noted: "Big data may be 99% irrelevant. Big data will not be used to find order in complexity but to confirm or refine what we already know."[37]

While I agree there is an opportunity in this space, it would require flipping some long-entrenched power dynamics.

Almost all devices for Parkinson's are designed to capture data relevant to clinicians. While understandable from the clinician's point of view, it overlooks the fact that the vast majority of trials and treatment strategies do not happen within the purview of the clinic.

Every day people with Parkinson's run trials on themselves. We constantly tweak our sleep schedules, medication, nutrition, hydration, stress and anxiety levels, temperature, and so much more, each of which have an effect on how our symptoms manifest. Tracking and optimizing all of these variables is nearly impossible. But if we had passive devices designed to give the user objective measures that they consider useful to help them track their disease and manage their symptoms, it could revolutionize how we manage and treat these diseases.

Getting there would require a radical redesign to how we deliver healthcare.[5] It would require a shift to a system focused on empowering patients to make their own decisions about their health. A system centered on the patient rather than the doctor.

I'll leave it to Sara once again to sum it all up: "The key is to find ways to measure things that help people make meaningful choices about issues that are important to them. Currently, the frenzy is to market products that measure things that are easy to quantify, regardless of whether they help people or not."

---

[5] Note that I have deliberately shifted the last discussion from technology to understand the disease (doubtful as currently conceived) to technology to help understand my fluctuations (achievable in the short term!). Most of the discussion in this book centers on "the disease" as a construct to "modify" (disease modification). While also critically important, we are not tackling in this book the important subject of how to improve day-to-day symptoms in individual patients (symptomatic therapies)

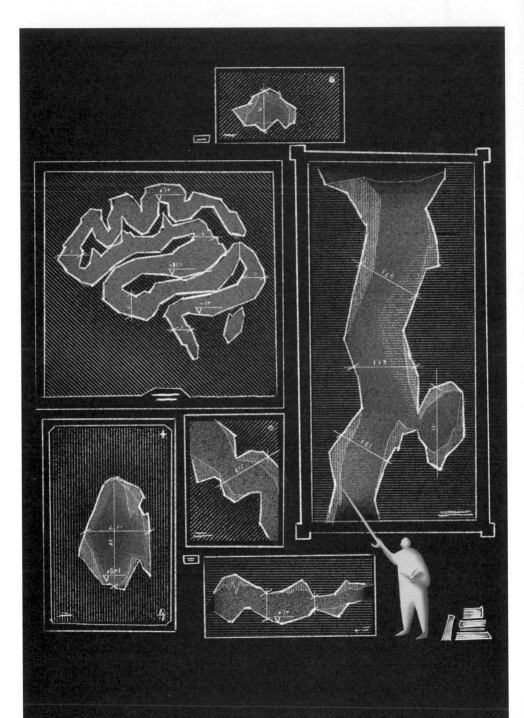

Chapter 8

Lessons from Oncology

There's always a story. It's all stories, really. The sun coming up every day is a story. Everything's got a story in it. Change the story, change the world.

Terry Pratchett

After taking the patient's history and completing a full examination, Dr. Smith summarizes his findings: "Based on my experience and the diagnostic criteria available, you have Disease X. We could support this diagnosis by Test Y, although my clinical impression should suffice. Because the progression of Disease X varies among patients, it is impossible to predict the speed of such progression for you. I suggest we start Treatment Z soon."

Dr. Smith was an oncologist delivering the diagnosis of breast cancer, circa 1970. The treatment he proposed was radical mastectomy, the standard of care for everyone with breast cancer. A future clinical trial, in 1981, would show that when radical mastectomy was compared with breast-preserving surgery, there was no difference in outcomes.[115] A similar proportion of patients survived in both arms.

From that landmark study, the approach to evaluating treatments for breast cancer changed forever. The hypothesis that breast cancer was a bad disease of the breast was rejected, replaced with the hypothesis that breast cancer represented several diseases, and that each might have a different set of biological drivers, unique courses, and require separate treatment approaches.

In the vignette above, Dr. Smith could have been a neurologist delivering the diagnosis of Parkinson's disease with Test Y being a measure of dopamine deficiency (DATscan) and Treatment Z, selegiline, a treatment that allows more dopamine to linger around in the synapse, circa 2005. Unlike the recalibration that began in oncology in the 1980s, when breast and other cancers started to be subdivided based on molecular markers, the approach to neurodegenerative disease has remained frozen in time, leading to the dubious record in medicine of accruing 146 failed attempts between 1998 and 2017 to develop a therapy to slow Alzheimer's.[116] In Parkinson's, since the late 1980s there have been 19 treatments with enormous promise reaching Phase 3, the last phase of development, without success (Figure 24).

In oncology, negative trials became opportunities to reconsider the approach to therapeutic development. In neurodegenerative diseases, negative trials have been viewed as artifacts of trial design and execution. We have kept on insisting that positive outcomes are within reach if only these studies are better designed and recruit patients at an earlier stage.

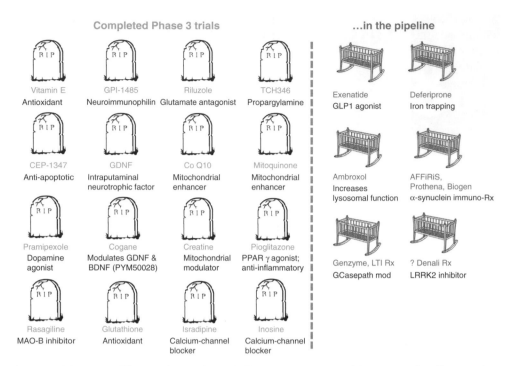

Figure 24 Disease-modifying trials in Parkinson's disease: consequence of the one-size-fits-all approach to treatment. Selected interventions that failed Phase 3 trials in Parkinson's disease are shown in tombstones. The trials "in the pipeline" follow the same 'one-drug-fits-all' approach. (Illustration by Tonya Hines, Glia Media).

Oncology is the biological mirror-image to neurodegeneration. In oncology, cells abnormally grow; in neurodegeneration, they abnormally age. Cancer was once viewed as a single, if heterogeneous, disease. Breast cancer was treated with radical mastectomy regardless of disease stage because it was believed that all forms were similarly aggressive and malignant.[117] In the 1950s and 1960s, the application of breast-conserving surgery ("quadrantectomy" or "lumpectomy") was widely believed to be inappropriate compared to radical surgery. Only as of the early 1980s, after a randomized clinical trial comparing these procedures demonstrated no difference in survival,[115,118] did researchers begin to consider breast cancer as a cluster of several diseases. Only then did they begin searching for its biological subtypes.

The last three decades of cancer research redefined cancer entirely, using a systems-biology approach to guide classification and disease-modifying treatment strategies. Under this paradigm for breast cancer, researchers arrived at a combination of nine histological types, which when associated with validated molecular markers, have yielded nearly 20 breast cancer subtypes, each with distinct survival curves and sensitivity to therapies.[119,120]

Unlike oncology, the field of neurodegenerative diseases does not have ready access to affected tissue to biopsy and study, which has contributed to the long dominance of clinical (and more recently, brain imaging) criteria for biomarker development. An oncologist examines several biomarkers in order to tailor a disease-modifying anticancer treatment for an individual based on the specific histologic type, the plausible genetic mutations, the presence of various receptors, and the anatomical spread. Only after these data are obtained is *a disease* identified and the best therapeutic cocktail determined. Such cocktail addresses known mechanisms and pre-empts plausible secondary mechanisms of cancer development *for that specific patient*.

The time has come to abandon the illusion that we can "cure Parkinson's disease" (or Alzheimer's). We can only cure one molecularly defined subtype of disease at a time, just as oncologists have done for many cancers over several decades.

The most important lesson from oncology may well be that nothing that is common to everyone with a disease can become universal targets for treating that disease. Precision medicine depends on understanding that which is different about an individual with a disease in relation to others with the same disease. It does not thrive on targeting whatever is common across everyone with that disease. We shall delve into this issue in the next chapter.

Commentary – Patients, Pigeonholes, and Open Science

There are people studying just (mitochondrial) bioenergetics or protein import or calcium, who don't really know much about the other aspects of mitochondria. That is a big challenge. We spend decades becoming specialists, but now we need to back up and work together so we can put the whole puzzle together.
Heidi McBride, interview for tmrwedition.com *on April 24, 2018*

Not only are neuroscientists missing out on valuable lessons from other disease fields as Alberto just described, but even within their own subspecialty there is potentially useful information that doesn't pass from one department to the next. How did we get to the point that researchers are so immersed in their silos that they don't even know what colleagues studying the same organelle are working on?

The problem is institutional. The incentive structure that guides each academic's career has created a system in which the goal is not to integrate knowledge but to extend each domain as far as it can go. This has produced fields of subspecialists with very few generalists capable of seeing and analyzing the bigger picture.

As Eric Kandel, nobel laureate and one of the most revered neuroscientists on the planet, told me: "Of course there is a danger that you get so narrow that you begin to lose the forest through the trees. You have to be careful; reductionism is useful in certain contexts and not useful in others. It is an approach; like all approaches it has strengths, but it also has limitations."

So where do we go from here? How can we get more people to see the forest? How can we nudge the motivating factors that drive science forward towards ones more closely aligned with the needs of society? Can we figure out how to reward researchers for working toward more ambitious goals than their next publication or grant?

Well, it's not going to happen overnight, but here are two policy changes that I believe every biomedical research center and institution should adopt to get us moving in the right direction.

1. Commit to Open Science

Open science means different things to different people, but basically it is an attempt to more closely align the motivating factors that drive science with the needs of society. Much of the open science movement is centered around how knowledge gets transferred from the lab to the public. The model we currently use to disseminate scientific knowledge is painfully slow. When a scientific discovery is made it usually takes years just to make it into academic journals. A broadly implemented open science mandate would ensure much more rapid spread of new knowledge.

Thankfully there is already a lot of movement in this direction and growing support from institutions and government agencies. Perhaps the biggest push for open science has been Plan S, an initiative that has garnered support from a number of national science academies and some major funders of science research. "The plan requires scientists and researchers who benefit from state-funded research organisations and institutions to publish their work in open repositories or in journals that are available to all by 2021."[1],121

---

[1] Open-access journals will need to undergo scrutiny of their business model. Most require that authors pay to publish, creating an inherent conflict of interest: their very survival depends on publishing. This has lowered the threshold for quality, with "junk science" entering the medical literature, risking misinformation and misguidance of future endeavors.

There is another group pushing an even more radical open science policy. In 2016, backed by a donation from philanthropist Larry Tanenbaum, the Montreal Neurological Institute at McGill University launched the Tanenbaum Open Science Institute (TOSI), becoming the first academic institution to formally adopt open science policies.

The unique part of their open science policy concerns intellectual property (IP) protection. Working with Professor Richard Gold, (founding Director of the Centre for Intellectual Property Policy at McGill University), TOSI took the bold step of removing the practice of IP protection, believing that the agreements and legal proceedings that arise as a result of patents are bottlenecks slowing drug development.

"Universities and colleges need to structure their relations with industry – and each other – around collaborations rather than IP," said Professor Gold in an article for the Centre for International Governance Innovation. "Removing IP from the equation not only reduces out-of-pocket expenses in personnel and patent applications, but also greatly improves the circulation of knowledge to firms and other researchers who can make the best use of it."[122]

Time will tell if open science can be broadly applied, but if nothing else we are long overdue for some experimenting with new models that have the potential to accelerate drug development.

2. Patient-Centered Research

I have been to dozens of biotech companies and academic labs where I was the first patient to ever walk through their doors. Far too many researchers only see the diseases they study under a microscope. The only way to get researchers to see what they should be striving for is for them to have regular contact with those stakeholders who have the most at stake.

This sentiment was summed up brilliantly in an interview I did with Dr. Jon Stamford, who was a neuroscientist studying Parkinson's disease when he himself was diagnosed with the disease.

> I think I perceived it very much as James Parkinson himself did, and in one of the great ironies of life, I studied at the London Hospital Medical College, which is where 200 or so years earlier James Parkinson himself studied and wrote his paper on The Shaking Palsy. I very much saw the disease as the diagram he used, that most people see, of the increasingly stooped figure with the shuffled walk. My research was very much preclinical. I didn't see patients. The first actual patient I saw was myself.
>
> Bizarrely, I couldn't figure it out on my own. I had been teaching Parkinson's to medical students for years and I couldn't recognize the symptoms in myself. I attributed the slowness and other symptoms I was experiencing to advancing middle age. I was almost accidentally diagnosed because I had a problem with my shoulder that turned out to be a frozen shoulder, one of the classical symptoms of PD. That, along with deteriorating handwriting, led to my diagnosis.

In another very illuminating part of our interview he remarked:

> I have absolute, unwavering faith (in basic science). I don't see any other route. But I don't think we should channel all funding into primary research. That is a significant part of it and where the major leaps are going to come from, but those decisions have to be informed by patient input. Patients have to lead the agenda and be able to say to scientists, 'These are my priorities and these are the things that need addressing.' The idea of scientists alone making the decisions about what they perceive to be Parkinson's is insane. If I think back to who I was before (my) diagnosis, I wouldn't trust myself to make those decisions.

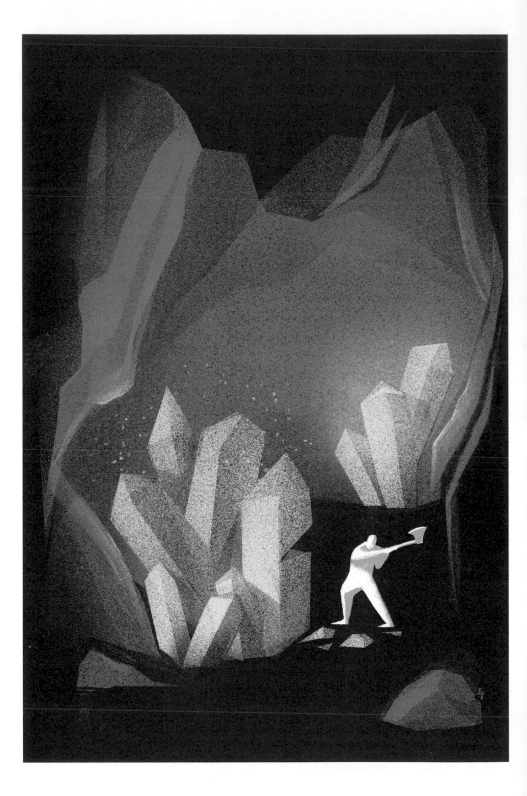

Symptomatic vs. Disease-Modifying Therapies

Medicine is not a science; it is empiricism founded on a network of blunders.
Emmet Densmore, How Nature Cures: Comprising a New System of Hygiene

Lumping "complex and heterogeneous" diseases into the single constructs of Parkinson's and Alzheimer's diseases has led to some successes on one front: the development of *symptomatic* therapies. These are treatments that can improve symptoms by targeting common denominators of a disease. In the case of Parkinson's, dopamine deficiency and norepinephrine deficiency are examples of eloquent common denominators. These neurotransmitters are produced at a lower rate than needed, resulting in some of the symptoms of Parkinson's. Dopamine deficiency, for instance, leads to slowness and stiffness. Norepinephrine deficiency contributes to depression and orthostatic hypotension (drops in blood pressure when standing). The strategies aimed at replacing dopamine include levodopa, a precursor of dopamine; dopamine agonists, which directly stimulate the dopamine receptors in the brain; and other agents that can be considered "fuel additives" because they make levodopa or dopamine last longer in the brain.

But what about the *disease*? That depends on whether we continue to view *the disease* as one multiheaded beast or reframe it as a collection of distinct animals, as we have argued in prior chapters. The former model assumes that all the clinical, genetic, and molecular variability are "modifiers" of a unifying pathological core, alpha-synuclein aggregates. Understanding a genetic "piece of the puzzle" has the capacity to inform the whole of the Parkinson's beast. The alternative model parses out Parkinson's *diseases* into distinct biological constructs that happen to share sufficient clinical and pathologic elements to be grouped under the same diagnostic umbrella.

The multiheaded-beast model behind Parkinson's disease assumes that a drug may act on most patients with Parkinson's because the mechanism of action is *sufficiently common* or *dominant* across all clinical subtypes. As mentioned above, dopamine replacement strategies have been well served as symptomatic treatments by this model because dopamine deficiency, from nigrostriatal neurodegeneration, is a dominant feature in all forms of Parkinson's disease. Dopamine replacement may be thought of as the energy that powers a city. If there is a problem with the grid that causes power outages in certain parts of the city, levodopa can be the generators used for rescue until we can correct the underlying electrical problem.

A widespread belief is that this model can work for disease modification if the intervention believed to be critical in Parkinson's as a whole is introduced *very early* (ideally at a *prodromal* or prediagnosis stage) in as many patients as possible.

Virtually all disease-modifying clinical trial efforts in Parkinson's and Alzheimer's diseases have to date been based on the concept that protein aggregation and molecular mechanisms linked to them represent the origin of these diseases in everyone. The results have been invariably disappointing (Table 5 in this chapter, Table 6 in the next). Many molecules found in low supply at autopsy have been interpreted as causal, including glutathione,[123] coenzyme Q10,[124] brain-derived neurotrophic factor,[125] glial cell-line-

Table 5 List of all reported Phase 3 clinical trials in Parkinson's disease of drugs once considered potential cures: invariably negative

Drug tested (drug or study name)	Mechanism of action	Parkinson's patients recruited
Tocopherol (vitamin E)[129]	Antioxidant	Early, drug-naïve
Coenzyme Q10 (CoQ10)[127]	Antioxidant; helps mitochondria	Early, drug-naïve
Mitoquinone (MitoQ)[130]	Antioxidant; helps mitochondria	Early, drug-naïve PD subjects
Creatine (LS1)[131]	Bioenergetic	Early, on any treatment
Pioglitazone (FS-ZONE)[132]	PPAR-γ agonist	Early on rasagiline or selegiline
Riluzole[133]	Glutamate antagonist	Early, drug-naïve
Selegiline (DATATOP and others)[129,134–136]	Antiapoptotic, GAPDH inhibitor, antioxidant	Early, drug-naïve
Rasagiline (ADAGIO)[137]	Antiapoptotic, GAPDH inhibitor, antioxidant	Early, drug-naïve
Pramipexole (PROUD)[138]	Antiapoptotic	Early, drug-naïve
Glutathione[139]	Antioxidant	Advanced
AAV2-Neurturin injected into SNpc and putamen[140]	Neurotrophic	Advanced
GDNF (Liatermin)[141]	Neurotrophic	Advanced
Paliroden[142]	Neurotrophic	Early, drug-naïve
PYM50028 (Cogane)[143]	Promotes release of GDNF and BDNF	Early, drug-naïve
Minocycline[144]	Anti-inflammatory, antiapoptotic	Early, drug-naïve
Immunophilin (GPI-1485)[145]	Antiapoptotic, possibly trophic	Mild to moderate
TCH346 (Omigapil)[146]	Antiapoptotic – GAPDH inhibitor	Early, drug-naïve
CEP-1347 (PRECEPT)[147]	Antiapoptotic – mixed-lineage kinase inhibitor	Early, drug-naïve

Interim analyses of two other interventions in clinical trials as of this writing (inosine and isradipine) demonstrated they were futile, but reports have not been published. Many other drugs have failed at earlier, less definitive phases of development. BDNF: brain-derived neurotrophic factor; GDNF: glial cell line-derived neurotrophic factor; GAPDH: glyceraldehyde 3-phosphate dehydrogenase; PPAR: peroxisome proliferator-activated receptor.

derived neurotrophic factor,[126] etc. There have been as many failed disease-modifying clinical trials as the molecules tested in them.[33]

For example, clinical trials of drugs that enhance mitochondrial function will continue to fail if they include a substantial number of patients for whom the assumed mitochondrial mechanism represents a byproduct or is minimally contributory. Cautionary tales for this particular example have been the large negative trials of coenzyme Q10[127] and creatine,[128] once held as the most promising strategies for disease modification in Parkinson's (most of the open-label studies that preceded the definitive trials were highly encouraging).

Under the "Parkinson's as a collection of distinct animals" model, selected mitochondrial enhancing strategies (e.g., favoring mitophagy or restoring electron transport chain activity) would be expected to succeed only in the subgroup of patients where mitochondrial dysfunction is *predominant and upstream.*

Commentary – What Pharma Wants vs. What Patients Want

The greater danger for most of us isn't that our aim is too high and we miss it, but that it is too low and we reach it.

Michelangelo

The pharmaceutical industry gets a bad rap... (Figure 25)

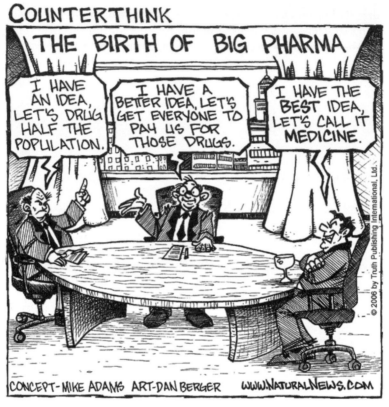

Figure 25 One of many examples of the reputation big pharma has. Though some may say that perception is reality, this ignores the vital role that only the pharmaceutical industry can play in the development of new therapies.

They are an easy scapegoat. Incredibly wealthy and powerful faceless entities that seem hell-bent on squeezing every penny they can out of desperate patients. While there are plenty of stories of unscrupulous practices from industry, they are not the bad guys that so many paint them to be.

I have visited dozens of pharmaceutical and biotech companies, often spending entire days touring their facilities and getting to know the people who work there. Most have the best of intentions and are sincerely trying to help individuals afflicted by the diseases they have devoted their lives to. They are constrained by market forces and investor interests, but they do what they can within those confines to bring therapies to market.

The important question is, what does it take to get something to market? What goal do they have in mind when they try to develop drugs that can alter the progression of Parkinson's or Alzheimer's or many other neurological conditions?

Well, it is actually pretty simple. Essentially they are trying to go from this…

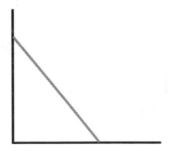

To this …

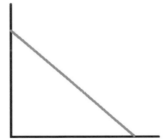

The sloped line represents the theoretical pace of degeneration for an average person diagnosed with a brain disease. It typically starts from the time of symptom onset to death or crippling disability. Pharma's goal is to develop a profitable therapy that can statistically lessen the steepness of the slope to an extent better than placebo. If they can demonstrate that, the stock price of the company would jump, huge bonuses would be given, and champagne bottles would pop all through the night in company offices around the world.

While this would certainly be welcome news to all, the celebrations coming from the patient community would be a little more subdued. Let me explain. (I'll use Parkinson's as my example because it's the one I know best, but similar things can be said about most degenerative brain diseases.)

One myth often told in the Parkinson's community is "you don't die from Parkinson's, you die with Parkinson's." This is bogus, especially for young-onset cases. A diagnosis of Parkinson's disease is a prolonged death sentence; a slow, grueling, drawn out death sentence. And while we may be given 15–25 years to live after the diagnosis (rough figure, stats vary), those aren't exactly 15–25 pleasant years.

One way of putting this is using quality of life (QOL) scales. Here is what a simplified QOL graph looks like for the average person diagnosed with Parkinson's disease.

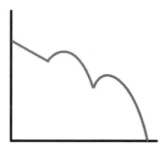

The first straight line represents the time from diagnosis to when one starts levodopa, the most effective symptomatic therapy we have. It is important to remember that each case is different, but it typically takes 1–3 years after diagnosis for a patient to start taking levodopa. After which there is a significant bump in quality of life. However, as the disease progresses, levodopa becomes less and less effective and has its own side effects that impact quality of life. This period can be anywhere from 2–10 years. This is generally followed by the "last line of defense," deep brain stimulation (DBS) surgery for those who qualify. DBS typically results in another bump in quality of life, but over time complications arise as the disease progresses, all sorts of motor and non-motor symptoms pop up that we do not have ways to properly manage, and eventually life itself becomes a daily struggle.

So, while all would welcome a 20% boost in the rate of decline, patients tend to have more ambitious goals in mind. For many of them success would look a little more like this …

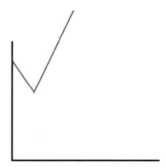

Though many would also settle for this …

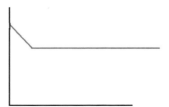

While some might say that we need to crawl before we can walk, we also need to ensure that we keep the end goal in mind. If the day ever comes when a drug does hit the mark, there will be far more champagne bottles being popped in industry offices around the world than in patient homes.

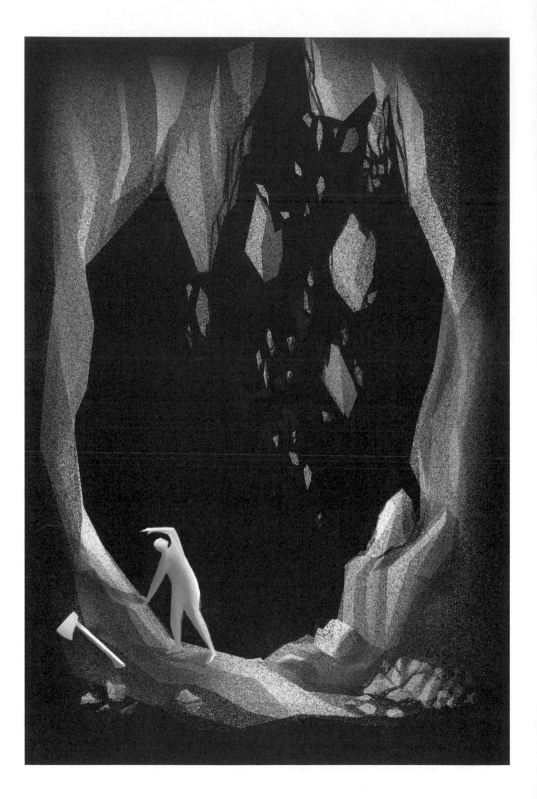

Chapter 10

The Hypothesis That Refuses to Die

The TV scientist who mutters sadly, "The experiment is a failure; we have failed to achieve what we had hoped for," is suffering mainly from a bad script writer. An experiment is never a failure solely because it fails to achieve predicted results. An experiment is a failure only when it also fails adequately to test the hypothesis in question, when the data it produces don't prove anything one way or another.

Robert M. Pirsig, Zen and the Art of the Motorcycle Maintenance An Inquiry into Values

Hypotheses are important generators of science. Every good research project is followed by at least one or more hypotheses for further research. A hypothesis is an idea built on prior studies that can be tested to demonstrate, for instance, an association between two or more variables or a beneficial effect of a treatment.

One of the major hypotheses generated in the twentieth century in the field of Alzheimer's disease was the "amyloid cascade hypothesis." This hypothesis argued that brain accumulation of beta-amyloid is the initial event in the chain of abnormalities leading to Alzheimer's disease. Amyloid misfolds first outside the cells, leading tau to be abnormally phosphorylated inside the cells, leading to degeneration of the neurons. This all happens in regions of the brain involved in memory, giving rise to what we can recognize at the bedside first as mild cognitive impairment, later as dementia. This cascade from amyloid to tau to neuronal death has been the hypothesis about the cause of Alzheimer's disease I grew up on in medical school.

Data from cell-based research has demonstrated that two enzymes called alpha-secretase and beta-secretase 1 (BACE1) act on a large membrane protein called amyloid precursor protein (APP) and make it a water-soluble product. Another, more complex enzyme, gamma-secretase, breaks one of the APP fragments into two smaller fragments, one of which is beta-amyloid. If the length of the beta-amyloid consists of 40 amino acids, it can be degraded; if it is 42 amino acids, it aggregates into, sequentially, monomers, oligomers, protofibrils, fibrils, and ultimately the beta-amyloid plaques considered the pathologic hallmark of Alzheimer's disease (the steps are in many ways analogous to those leading to the formation of Lewy bodies in Parkinson's disease).

The full hypothesis posits that the 42-amino-acid beta-amyloid becomes the "cradle" from which tau gets to be attached with too many phosphates or "phosphorylated." From there, it disrupts the structure of the axons, the elongated parts of the neurons, turning them into neurofibrillary tangles (Figure 26).

The amyloid hypothesis produced moments of rampant excitement, similar to those that formed what we could have termed the "alpha-synuclein cascade hypothesis." Like the Contursi effect for Parkinson's, the field of Alzheimer's research was shaped by the discovery of autosomal dominant mutations in the *APP* gene, as well as that of other genes (*PSEN1* and *PSEN2*).

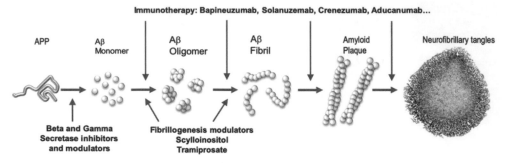

Figure 26 Amyloid cascade hypothesis in Alzheimer's disease and targets of treatments examined in clinical trials. Cell-based studies in animal models have identified these sequential steps in amyloid misfolding into plaques (outside of neurons) and the facilitation of tau phosphorylation into neurofibrillary tangles (inside the neurons). The stages mirror the steps in protein misfolding and aggregation outlined earlier as part of the formation of Lewy bodies in Parkinson's disease. To emphasize such analogy, the images for each stage are borrowed from those presented in Chapter 5 – appearance of alpha-synuclein and amyloid intermediaries actually differ but the overall steps are similar. (Illustration by Tonya Hines, Glia Media.)

In people with these mutations, beta-amyloid production went into overdrive, leading to early and severe dementia. And like *SNCA* mutations over-express alpha-synuclein and cause Parkinson's disease, *APP* mutations over-express beta-amyloid and cause Alzheimer's disease. Beta-amyloid became the cause of Alzheimer's in everyone with dementia of Alzheimer's type.

This hypothesis has had enormous influence. Every step between the formation of the 42-amino acid beta-amyloid and the creation of the beta-amyloid plaque has been the source of intense research from the late twentieth century onward. The National Institutes of Health's annual budget for Alzheimer's, largely centered on antiamyloid strategies, reached $2.3 billion in 2019, more than 5% of NIH's overall budget (Figure 27). The ambition for the increased funding, as dictated by the Department of Health and Human Services, NIH's parent department, is to "prevent and effectively treat Alzheimer's disease by 2025."

Preventing and treating a disease within the next five years requires knowing that disease very well today so that we can anticipate which tools to use. The allure of the amyloid hypothesis is that if any step of the process from amyloid aggregation to tau hyperphosphorylation could be blocked, we could stop the progression of Alzheimer's disease.

But how has this hypothesis fared so far? The war against anti-beta-amyloid has been one of attrition (Table 6). To date, over 20 drugs have been tried in Phase 3, the most advanced stage of development for any molecule of therapeutic promise. Every single one of them has failed to prove any benefit in clinical trials and a good chunk of the data suggests the targeting of amyloid can backfire.

This is important to emphasize: most of these studies demonstrated that the experimental intervention accomplished exactly what was intended. That is, the brain concentration of beta-amyloid was reduced, as measured by assays in the spinal fluid, brain imaging techniques, or a combination of both. So "target engagement," the ability of the drug to act in the designed manner, was achieved. Yet the results were either nil or worse.

Not only have all these trials been negative, but in nearly 40% of them the active-treatment arm worsened compared to the placebo arm, either because of deterioration in cognition, acceleration of brain atrophy, or both.

It is remarkable that a hypothesis so badly bruised continues to be tested time and again. How do we explain these failures and continue preserving the life of the amyloid hypothesis?

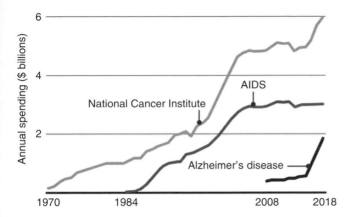

Figure 27 **Funding for Alzheimer's is up**. The National Institutes of Health (NIH) has ramped up funding for only three specific disease priorities: cancer, AIDS, and, most recently, Alzheimer's (Data from N. Desai/Science; (NIH Appropriations Data, Office of Aids Research. NIH RCDC. Published in Science 361:838, 2018 (DOI: 10.1126/SCIENCE.361.6405.838).[148] Reprinted with permission from *Science*.

In part, this is the product of America's low-risk approach to funding research. The National Institutes of Health has not funded exploratory, non-hypothesis-based studies, and therefore a bias exists for a continued "testing" of a hypothesis that is widely accepted.

A poignant summary of the experience of clinical trials for Alzheimer's disease in 2018, the last year for which full data are available, was summarized by David Knopman, an expert on Alzheimer's at the Mayo Clinic, in one page:[150]

- Crenezumab[151] and solanezumab[76] reduced amyloid burden as expected but induced no cognitive changes: this means the next study should examine the effect of higher doses.
- Verubecestat[152] reduced amyloid burden as expected but worsened cognitive function and accelerated brain atrophy: this means the next study should examine the effect of lower doses.

Although Knopman admitted that "something is wrong with the amyloid hypothesis" and "one must question whether reduction of beta-amyloid levels is the wrong therapeutic strategy,"[150] he agreed with the conclusions of the authors of these trials, namely that the issue was one of incorrect dosage. The drugs may not have worked well enough when dosed too low (crenezumab and solanezumab) or worked too well when dosed too high (verubecestat)!

Two other alibis continue giving oxygen to the amyloid hypothesis. The first is that targeting at the *prodromal* stage is the clear solution because it is the absolute earliest time to act and doing so will finally prove that antiamyloid strategies can work. The second is that antiamyloid therapies need a little extra help: they should be combined with some other therapies in what is referred to as the "cocktail approach."

The news coverage of the latest string of failures has added yet another explanation for the failures: *once symptoms appear it is already too late*.[1] If the amyloid hypothesis cannot

---

[1] Let us imagine what the world of cancer treatment might look like if oncologists would have concluded from their early clinical-trial disappointments, as neurologists do with theirs, that once any symptoms of cancer appear, it may be too late. Or that the negative outcomes of the trials are to always be attributed to the imperfections of the trials rather than the hypotheses supporting them.

Table 6 The 35 Phase 2 and Phase 3 randomized clinical trials of antiamyloid drugs for Alzheimer's disease

Drug, Year	Mechanism	Population	Phase	TE	Outcome
AN-1792, 2002	Aβ antigen	Mild-mod AD	2	Y	No change, toxic
Tramiprosate, 2007	Aβ aggregation inhibitor	Mild-mod AD	3	Y	No change
Tarenflurbil, 2009	γ-Secretase modulator	Mild AD	3	N	Worse globally
Scyllo-inositol, 2009	Aβ aggregation inhibitor	Mild-mod AD	2	Y	Increase mortality
Begacestat, 2010	γ-Secretase inhibitor	Mild-mod AD	2	N	No change, toxic
Ponezumab, 2011	Anti-Aβ antibody	Mild-mod AD	2	N	No change
Semagacestat, 2011	γ-Secretase inhibitor	Mild-mod AD	3	Y	Worse cognition, toxic
Bapineuzumab, 2012	Anti-Aβ antibody	Mild-mod AD	3	N	No change
Avagacestat, 2012	γ-Secretase inhibitor	Mild-mod AD	2	Y	Worse cognition
Avagacestat, 2012	γ-Secretase inhibitor	Prodromal AD	2	Y	Worse cognition, atrophy
Solanezumab, 2013	Anti-Aβ antibody	Mild-mod AD	3	Y	No change
Vanutide, 2013	Aβ antigen	Mild-mod AD	2	N	No change
Immunoglobulin, 2013	Anti-Aβ antibody	Mild-mod AD	3	N	No change
LY2886721, 2013	β-Secretase inhibitor	Mild-mod AD	2	Y	No change, toxic
AZD3839, 2013	β-Secretase inhibitor	Healthy	1	NR	Toxic; unpublished
Affitope AD02, 2014	Aβ antigen	Early AD	2	NR	Worse cognition
CAD106, 2014	Aβ antigen	Mild AD	2	Y	Worse cognition, atrophy
PBT2, 2014	Aβ aggregation inhibitor	Prodromal AD	2	N	No change
Crenezumab, 2014	Anti-Aβ antibody	Mild-mod AD	2	Y	No change

Table 6 (cont.)

Drug, Year	Mechanism	Population	Phase	TE	Outcome
Gantenerumab, 2014	Anti-Aβ antibody	Prodromal AD	2	Y	No change
Gantenerumab, 2014	Anti-Aβ antibody	Mild AD	2	Y	No change
Solanezumab, 2016	Anti-Aβ antibody	Mild AD	3	Y	No change
Solanezumab, 2016	Anti-Aβ antibody	Prodromal AD	3	NR	Terminated, unpublished
Verubecestat, 2016	BACE inhibitor	Mild-mod AD	3	Y	Worse atrophy
Verubecestat, 2018	BACE inhibitor	Prodromal AD	3	Y	Worse cognition
Atabecestat, 2018	BACE inhibitor	Mild AD	3	Y	No change
Lanabecestat, 2018	BACE inhibitor	Mild AD	3	Y	Terminated, worse cognition
Crenezumab, 2018	Anti-Aβ antibody	Mild-mod AD	2	Y	No change
Solanezumab, 2018	Anti-Aβ antibody	Mild AD	3	N	No change
Verubecestat, 2018	BACE inhibitor	Mild-mod AD	3	Y	Worse cognition
Verubecestat, 2018	BACE inhibitor	Prodromal AD	3	Y	Worse cognition
Aducanumab, 2019 (x2)	Anti-Aβ antibody	Mild AD	3	Y	Benefit announced* (1/2)
Lanabecestat, 2019 (x2)	BACE inhibitor	Mild AD	3	Y	No change (2/2)

AD, Alzheimer's disease. Aβ, beta-amyloid; NR: not reported. TE: target engagement (met in 67% of trials). Distribution of effects: null, 59%, worse in active arm, 38%; proportion of worsening in prodromal AD, 50%. *At press time, the interim negative results for one of the two Aducanumab trials were retracted by Biogen in an announcement to investors and the public. This table was updated and modified from from Panza and colleagues (*Nat Rev Neurol.* 2019 Feb;15(2):73–88])[149] The last two rows represent two trials each.

be rejected after negative upon negative trial then it must be proven at a time patients are not yet patients. Knopman himself added this note of caution to his summary of the clinical trial experience of 2018: "…prodromal Alzheimer's disease could represent a disease stage in which neurodegeneration is still too advanced for this treatment to be effective."[150]

In fact, six trials of selected antiamyloid therapies have been conducted on "prodromal" cohorts, that is, individuals with symptoms of mild cognitive impairment not fulfilling criteria for dementia. Three of these showed not just a null effect but *deterioration* in the treated arm compared with the placebo arm. Treated patients progressed more rapidly from cognitive impairment to dementia and, when reported, brain atrophy accelerated.

Clinical trialists often worry that negative results in a trial reflect a lower number of patients recruited, an insufficient sample size than would have been necessary to demonstrate the putative benefit of the intervention tested. This is referred to by statisticians as a "type 2 error." In these trials, however, the problem is not one of inadequate statistical power to be resolved by recruiting more patients into future trials. The problem is that despite adequate target engagement the actual effect is in the opposite direction to that which was hypothesized. These antiamyloid drugs washed the brain off amyloid, as they were designed to do, but patients worsened.

In the days following the initial drafting of this chapter, on March 21, 2019, Biogen announced it would discontinue the two concurrent Phase 3 trials of aducanumab. The analysis of an independent data-monitoring committee determined these trials were unlikely to meet the predefined primary efficacy endpoint. The scenario dramatically changed when we were working on the final edits of this book. On October 22, 2019, as part of its Third Quarter Financial Results and Business Update, Biogen notified investors and the public that the data then "suggested a different possible outcome than that predicted by the futility analysis."[153] The company indicated plans to file an application to the FDA in early 2020 to gain regulatory approval for aducanumab to reduce clinical decline in Alzheimer's disease.

None of the data from the futility analyses conducted in March 2019 was made available during the October 2019 analysis; we only have access to the company's summary of the revised analysis. The document acknowledges that the trials were in fact not discontinued in March but rather enlarged from 1,748 patients to a total of 2,066 subjects, counting those completing the 18-month protocol. These 318 additional patients, a 15% increase in sample size, were preferentially allocated to the high-dose arm, presumably without breaking the double-blind design. With greater statistical power, it was announced that one of the two clinical trials, *EMERGE*, met the prespecified primary endpoint and all secondary endpoints. Amyloid was reduced and cognitive function improved according to the global scores of two separate scales.

The news release by Biogen explained the turn-around as a fortunate convergence of multiple factors: "greater exposure to aducanumab in the larger dataset, including data on a greater number of patients, a longer average duration of exposure to high dose, the timing of protocol amendments that allowed a greater proportion of patients to receive high dose, and the timing and prespecified criteria of the futility analysis." That is, getting over the hump required the right timing, the right dosage, and the right analysis – which fewer than 2,000 patients could not deliver.

A public presentation and scrutiny of the data is pending as of press time. Meanwhile, the Biogen stock value jumped nearly 40% in the days following the announcement and was predicted to double in the months ahead.

What may be the most important development in neuroscience in decades was not to be welcomed by standing ovation at a scientific meeting or scrutinized in the peer-reviewed literature, but by the sanitized report to investors created for a corporate board meeting. The ramifications of this decision and the outcome of the FDA review that will follow may span beyond the life of millions at stake, catapulting neurology into a new era or setting it back years.

Commentary – Methodological Madness

The discovery of instances which confirm a theory means very little if we have not tried, and failed, to discover refutations. For if we are uncritical we shall always find what we want: we shall look for, and find, confirmation, and we shall look away from, and not see, whatever might be dangerous to our pet theories. In this way it is only too easy to obtain what appears to be overwhelming evidence in favour of a theory which, if approached critically, would have been refuted.

Karl Popper, The Poverty of Historicism

One of the foundational pillars on which the scientific method stands is that the beliefs of science must be falsifiable. That is, for a hypothesis to be accepted it must prove itself able to withstand rigorous experiments designed to prove it wrong.

Science in neurodegeneration seems to have skipped that lesson.

One of the speakers at the Revision vs. Reconstruction conference that Alberto will mention in Chapter 13 was Professor Virginia Lee. Professor Lee is one of the most revered figures in the field. She has arguably done as much to advance our hypotheses around protein aggregation as anyone and just received the $3 million Breakthrough Prize in Life Science for doing so. After her talk I went to the microphone and asked what I thought was a pretty simple, almost naïve question: "What experiments do we need to run to disprove the hypothesis that alpha-synuclein aggregation is the main cause of Parkinson's disease?"

What struck me as odd was not only the response that I got from her, which was wavering and did not directly address the question, but the praise that I received afterwards from several notable scientists in attendance for just posing the question.

It was similar to what I got while attending a conference in the summer of 2018 called, simply enough, Synuclein. At that conference over 100 scientists from around the world came together on the Swiss shore of Lake Geneva overlooking the French Alps to spend three days talking about nothing else but alpha-synuclein. Afterwards I posted a blog entry that included the following, "You might think that three days of discussion from over one hundred experts on a single protein must mean we understand it pretty well. Unfortunately, what was clear from all the talks was just how little we know about this basic building block of biology and its role in disease. There are still a lot of simple questions that nobody can definitively answer: What is the normal function of synuclein? How does the misfolding begin? Is the clumping part of the cells' defense mechanisms? How does it actually lead to the symptoms we see? Why have we not been able to develop biomarkers and imaging agents to monitor the spread of these clumps and disease progression?"

During that conference I asked one of the panels, "What is the best evidence we have that synuclein aggregates are an effect of having the disease rather than a cause?" I was met mostly with a mix of befuddlement and murmured sneering, but did get some sincere responses basically saying, "we don't really have any."

For two decades now alpha-synuclein has been one of the strongest clues we have had as to what is going wrong in Parkinson's. Almost everyone diagnosed with this disease is found to have clumps of this protein accumulating in their brains, so it seems reasonable to believe that it has something to do with the disease. As a result, as of this writing, there are nine therapies targeting alpha-synuclein being tested in humans, with dozens more in various stages of preclinical development.

All that money being poured into this target has driven many groups to look for any evidence that can validate the link between protein aggregates and disease. There are few if any incentives in place for running experiments designed to poke holes in this theory, or simply investigate alternative explanations for why these clumps are there. For all we know the relationship between protein aggregation and degenerative brain diseases could be similar to that of tornadoes and trees. Tornadoes tend to uproot trees and leave a trail of them in their wake, but no amount of research into the nature of fallen trees will help us avoid or prevent tornadoes.

Groucho Marx famously quipped that, "Politics is the art of looking for trouble, finding it everywhere, diagnosing it incorrectly and applying the wrong remedies." Sounds to me like he could just as easily be describing the state of neuroscience today. Protein aggregation has come to dominate our attempts to tackle these diseases to such an extent that any evidence of something having even the slightest effect on protein buildups is enough to get studies accepted into high-ranking journals.

A perfect example of this is an article published in the *Proceedings of the National Academy of Science*, titled "β-Amyloid accumulation in the human brain after one night of sleep deprivation."[159] It attracted wide media attention. Here is the summary: 20 healthy people ranging from 22 to 72 years of age were tested with a PET scan to measure brain beta-amyloid after a night of good sleep and after a night of sleep deprivation (being awake for about 31 hours). Compared with the rested night, the night of sleep deprivation led to a 5% increase in beta-amyloid in several brain regions, including the thalamus and hippocampus.

There are two possible conclusions.

The first generated eye-grabbing headlines because it is aligned with the field's toxic-amyloid narrative: "Lighting the Fire – Sleep deprivation can cause Alzheimer's disease."

The second never saw the light of day: "Brain Defense – Beta-amyloid acutely increases in response to sleep deprivation."

There is nothing in the data shown by the investigators that questions the second conclusion. But amyloid causes Alzheimer's as fallen trees cause the tornadoes.

The investigators did not examine whether the increase in beta-amyloid in the study participants would subside after a night of rest. This is the likeliest scenario since amyloid levels fluctuate during sleep via the glymphatic system.[160] Science calls for experiments to disprove the hypothesis that beta-amyloid aggregation is the main cause of Alzheimer's disease and alpha-synuclein aggregation of Parkinson's disease. But why ruin a good story?

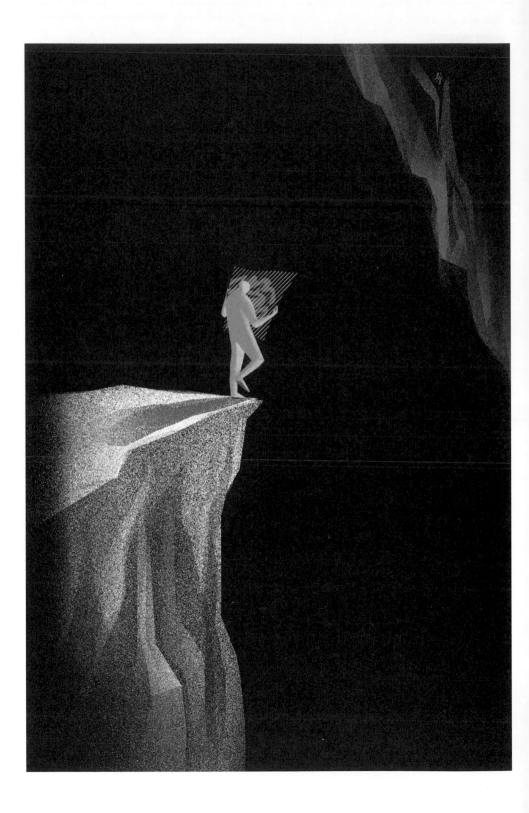

Chapter 11
Our Living Dissonance

We do not see things as they are, we see things as we are.

This quote is of unknown origin, variously attributed to Anaïs Nin, Babylonian Talmud, Immanuel Kant, G. T. W. Patrick, H. M. Tomlinson, Steven Covey, and anonymous

Mutations in the alpha-synuclein gene cause Parkinson's disease. In patients with these mutations, alpha-synuclein aggregate and literally choke the neurons to death.

Parkinson's is a collection of many genetic and non-genetic diseases that accumulate alpha-synuclein. Because alpha-synuclein gene mutations cause Parkinson's, and because clumps of it are found in almost every brain of individuals diagnosed with Parkinson's, alpha-synuclein aggregation must be the universal cause of Parkinson's disease.

Parkinson's disease is a collection of many diseases. Alpha-synuclein is a promising biomarker of Parkinson's disease.

And that sums up our cognitive dissonance.

It may seem subtle, but we can switch effortlessly between accepting Parkinson's *disease* and Parkinson's *diseases*. We can accept that each of these opposite tenets is true. It almost seems as if the acceptance of one tenet, Parkinson's as the sum of its parts, does not invalidate the other, Parkinson's as a collection of biologically distinct entities.

Alpha-synuclein is clearly causal in Parkinson's disease due to alpha-synuclein mutations and multiplications. These patients should be the only plausible candidates for ongoing clinical trials of antibody-based therapies against alpha-synuclein aggregates. Instead, these trials are enrolling everyone with a clinical diagnosis of Parkinson's disease, 99.9% of whom are unlikely to harbor an alpha-synuclein gene mutation.

How do we continue to live with this dissonance? By equal parts meticulous reasoning and pragmatism. Let me explain.

First, let's delve into the reasoning influence. This is how the main argument goes for accepting the dissonance: *the concept of Parkinson's as many diseases doesn't discount a potential important role for alpha-synuclein in many of them, not just the genetic forms*. The type and distribution of alpha-synuclein are so similar in cases with vs. without alpha-synuclein mutations that alpha-synuclein cannot be merely a bystander or just play a protective role. Also, we need to keep an open mind that the genetic forms can also inform us about important potential causal mechanisms in patients who lack the genetic variations.

This reasoning accepts the reality of Parkinson's *diseases,* but with a great deal of overlap between diseases (as in model C, in Figure 28). They share so much as to ultimately be more

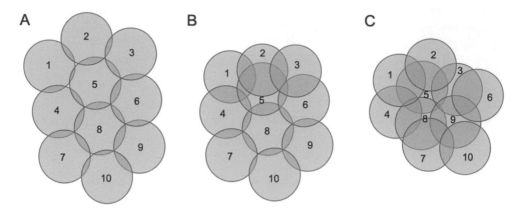

Figure 28 Conceptual models of Parkinson *diseases* (each numbered circle represents *a disease*, a biological entity). In model A, while the diseases are related, they are mostly unique; some biological elements are shared but most are not. In model B, some diseases are more biologically related than others. In model C, all diseases bear a strong relationship to one another and their "uniqueness" is mostly theoretical: for instance, treatment for Disease 5 could benefit from treatments designed for Diseases 1, 2, 3, 4 and 8. In this model, the separation of diseases bears little practical relevance when considering treatment approaches.

alike than distinct. We suspect that what might work therapeutically in one type could well work on others.

Our reductionist nature has trained us to apply rules of convergence to a range of observations. If we learned that Disease 1 is generated by an excessive accumulation of alpha-synuclein, then over-production or under-degradation of alpha-synuclein must also be a problem for Diseases 2 through 10. Hence, a treatment designed with Disease 1 in mind could work for most diseases.

How about the practical aspects of considering Parkinson's as one and many diseases at once? This argument is divided into two parts. The first is economic. Dividing Parkinson's into many diseases does away with the hope that a treatment will have an impact on the lives of most patients, especially those without any known cause. For those of us involved in clinical trials, we always think: *we have to instill hope in everyone with Parkinson's each time we invest in a clinical trial.*

The other aspect is cultural. We have an ingrained distrust of the validity of negative trials.

The very training of neurologists nurtures intellectual skepticism. While this is healthy in reviewing data from all studies, skepticism also extends into permanently questioning whether negative clinical trials are truly accurate or whether they may represent "false negatives." A fragment of an interview that Ben conducted for his website with Professor J. Timothy Greenamyre, chief of movement disorders and director of the Pittsburgh Institute for Neurodegenerative Diseases, illustrates this point:

Question: *If our current approaches fail, would that mean that our basic assumptions of this disease are wrong, or would we just have to find new ways of testing our assumptions?*

Answer: *I think the latter. I learned from a great neurologist that clinical trials are a terrible way to test a scientific hypothesis. There are so many reasons why a clinical trial can fail that have nothing to do with the basic science behind the trial. The dose could be wrong, the drug might not be hitting the target effectively, etc. Unfortunately, when a trial fails it could lead to the death of that target because investors will be more hesitant to put money into similar drugs for the same target.*

This response is the one most neurologists have endorsed from time immemorial. The assumptions about disease are well established; the methods to test them, however, are imperfect. The implication is that all therapies developed based on accepted approaches are inherently effective. As such, a positive trial confirms our hypothesis; a negative trial must be questioned and is unlikely to reject the hypothesis that inspired it.

While imperfect, there is no method of higher caliber than a randomized clinical trial to test hypotheses of therapeutic significance. There has to be a time when negative trials must be understood as "true negatives" or "correct failures," allowing for the hypothesis tested to be appropriately rejected or reconfigured.

We cannot have it both ways with diseases of brain aging. We cannot accept the opposing tenets that Parkinson's is many diseases and that a given therapeutic approach stands a chance to slow the progression of Parkinson's (meaning the entire spectrum).

We can be pragmatic. In the short term, we can focus on the treatment of genetic forms of Parkinson's, such as GBA-enhancing therapies for Parkinson's disease patients with *GBA* mutations or LRRK2 inhibitors for Parkinson's disease patients with *LRRK2* mutations. The cultural change we need is to accept that success in either of these endeavors will not predict response in *idiopathic* Parkinson's disease, that is, everyone else without *GBA* or *LRRK2* mutations.

Walking the talk of Parkinson's as many diseases is admittedly unsexy. Accepting that the first success in disease modification for Parkinson's (as for just about any other neurodegenerative diseases) will likely apply to 1% or 2% of patients – or perhaps as many as 5% – is not attractive to payors, to foundations, to the NIH, or to patients. But it is our best hope if we want to start accruing successes in the 2020s and beyond.

Commentary – Genetic Dissonance?

In decades of study, genetics has become more rather than less complex. Mendel knew exactly what a gene was, what it did, and how it interacted with other genes. That certainly is not true today. Genetic manipulation or targeted vaccines are not going to be "magic bullets". Complexity will work against genetic treatment: what succeeds for one race, family, or type of disease may very well have no action outside that context.

Angela Scheuerle, Limits of the Genetic Revolution, 2001[154]

I have a mutation in my *GBA* gene. *GBA* mutations are known to elevate one's risk for Parkinson's disease, so most researchers and doctors I have spoken to assume that my Parkinson's is caused by my *GBA* mutation. Many of them have suggested to me that I sign up for one of the ongoing trials targeting this mutation.

This sounds like very good news. These GBA-targeted trials are among the most promising trials in all of neurology. For many they represent our best hope for a proof-of-concept precision therapy for neurodegeneration. As a result, significant resources are now pouring into this target.

However, as Ziv Gan-Or, a neurogeneticist and professor at McGill University, pointed out to me, genetics can only tell us so much about this disease. "We have measured heritability and determined the overall contribution of all genetic risk factors. That number is around 30%, which means most factors are not genetic."

So at best, even if we had a perfect understanding of all the genetic variables that went into my disease (which most would suspect includes much more than just my *GBA* mutation), we would still not be able to account for 70% of the reason why I have this disease.

Even more disconcerting is this quote from my interview with Professor Clemens Scherzer, Associate Professor of Neurology at Harvard Medical School, for an article I wrote for the *Journal of Parkinson's* blog:

> *Disease progression, not susceptibility to disease, is the key determinant of patients' well-being. How can we stop or prevent the disease from progressing instead of waiting and playing catch-up? Identifying the genetic drivers of disease progression – not susceptibility – in patients with PD will allow (for) slowing the progression and possibly prevent disabling complications such as dementia from ever occurring.*
>
> *This will require a paradigm shift in genetics from susceptibility genetics to prognosis genetics. Almost all of what we know about the genetics of Parkinson's disease today relates exclusively to susceptibility for developing the disease, not progression. For example, we know much about genetic loci that increase the risk of healthy people to develop Parkinson's in the future. This might lead to primary preventive therapies, but this is a very long-term goal in the absence of biomarkers. Patients with Parkinson's disease already have Parkinson's. The question is no longer about primary prevention, but preventing progression. The key question for slowing their progression is what are the progression loci, not susceptibility loci, and how can we target them.*
>
> *The reason (no one has done this yet) is that one needs deeply phenotyped longitudinal patient cohorts to do this fundamental experiment. That would require a lot of hard work over a long period of time and substantial amounts of funding as we would need to follow thousands of patients for many years. We are currently looking at 5,000 patients over the course of 12 years in the International Genetics of Parkinson's Disease*

Progression (IGPP) Consortium, but that's just the beginning. Tens of thousands would be needed.

All susceptibility genetics/GWAS studies just look at shallow data (diagnosis, age, sex) from poorly characterized patients with no longitudinal follow-up. It's the low-hanging fruit, but not necessarily most pertinent to patients. (GWAS: genome-wide association studies)

So, not only can genetics not explain my Parkinson's disease, but we may have been looking at the wrong set of genetic markers all along. And, as if things weren't murky enough, here is how Harvard Professor and Cancer Geneticist John Quackenbush explained one more aspect of genetics to me that further complicates things:

Genes and genetic variants group together into communities, and those communities tend to be associated with specific functions within cells. This moves us from an old model in which a single genetic variation might influence a single gene and takes us to a model in which a group of genetic variants could not just shift a particular gene, but could actually change how a cell functions. This has allowed us to move from just looking at one variant, one trait, to examining families of variants that increase the likelihood of a person being tall or developing a disease like Parkinson's.[Mar 19, 2018]

So to sum up my skepticism around these genetic targets:

1. Genetics can only explain a fraction of the reason why someone goes on to develop a form of Parkinson's.
2. The markers we have been looking at might not even be the markers most relevant to one's disease.
3. Very few genes can be studied or targeted in isolation, and only by understanding the complex network of genes within which they reside can we truly, purposefully understand and intervene.

Yet despite all of these concerns, there is near consensus in the field that GBA-related Parkinson's constitutes our best bet for a disease-modifying therapy in a subset of the Parkinson's population. While I hope it truly is as promising as everyone seems to believe, I cannot help but wonder if we are underestimating the problem yet again.

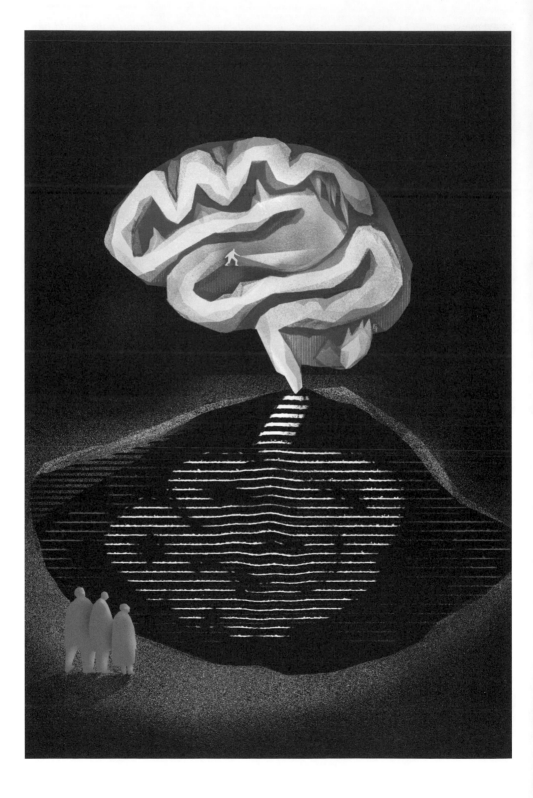

Chapter 12

The Scientific and Lay Narratives

It ain't what you don't know that gets you into trouble. It's what you know for sure that just ain't so.

Mark Twain

An editorial perfectly timed as we approached the final work on this book was published in the October 2019 issue of *Lancet Neurology*. With the title, "Re-aligning scientific and lay narratives of Alzheimer's disease," several Alzheimer's investigators pointed out a discrepancy between the narratives circulated among Alzheimer's patient advocates and those in academic circles.[155] The advocates' narrative centers around the belief that each case of Alzheimer's is its own unique disease; the scientific narrative, while acknowledging the heterogeneity, is based on a "theory of everything," the overarching path to Alzheimer's that can be generally applied to all cases.

That second narrative, in part because of the esteemed researchers behind it, attracts the lion's share of funding. It portrays neuroscience as being on the brink of treatments to slow down Alzheimer's. All that is needed is larger, more resource-intensive studies into what is being done to address everyone's Alzheimer's disease.

But the major misalignment the authors of this piece worry about is summarized in these two paragraphs:

A substantial body of biological, genetic, and epidemiological evidence indicates that amyloid deposition in the brain (brain amyloidosis) is an early event in the disease course, that amyloid is often followed by aggregation and spread of hyperphosphorylated tau, and that this is followed by synaptic dysfunction, neuronal loss, cognitive dysfunction, and finally progression to dementia. Importantly, the phase when biological events (amyloid and tau deposition) are detectable by imaging or CSF markers in the absence of cognitive dysfunction can last up to 20 years, and 20 to 30% of healthy individuals aged 65 years and over have substantial amounts of amyloid in their brain.

The evidence associating amyloid deposition with adverse cognitive outcomes is mounting, such that scientists have re-conceptualized Alzheimer's disease as a state that comprises primarily brain amyloidosis and tauopathy, irrespective of cognitive symptoms. This operational framework (also known as A/T/N, from the biological markers of amyloidosis, tauopathy, and neurodegeneration) is a key enabler to identify asymptomatic persons who might be on the way to develop dementia and enroll them in clinical trials of anti-amyloid or anti-tau drugs to prevent or delay cognitive impairment. However, this new framework also stipulates that, for instance, a 70-year-old person with no memory symptoms, normal cognitive performance, and no disability, but who has an abnormal PET or CSF amyloid test, is on the Alzheimer's disease continuum.

According to the scientific narrative, everything converges on amyloid and tau. A normal person with evidence of amyloid and tau in their central nervous system is on the "Alzheimer's continuum." The lay narrative does not include a state of normal memory with "brain amyloidosis" but centers instead on progressive forgetfulness, leading to severe and disabling loss of self-sufficiency.

The authors therefore proposed that it may be possible to "realign" these narratives by reframing brain amyloidosis in normal individuals as a state of "risk for neurode-generative dementia," just as hypertension came to be seen as a risk for developing cardiovascular disease. This opens the door for "more research on amyloid-lowering agents." Since hypertension eventually became "a disease" in its own right, so could brain amyloidosis.

The analogy with hypertension is worth reviewing. The National Heart Institute funded the largest cohort study in history in 1948 to follow 5,209 residents of the city of Framingham, in Massachusetts, recruited between the ages of 30 and 62 with no history of heart attack or stroke. One of the key findings was that elevated blood pressure was a common and powerful predisposing factor for stroke, coronary disease, cardiac failure and peripheral artery disease, increasing by two- to threefold the risk of one or more of these atherosclerotic complications.[156] However the causal link between hypertension and cardiovascular disease was controversial until 1967, when another large trial (the VACS, for Veterans Administration Cooperative Study) determined that the combination of hydrochlorothiazide, reserpine, and hydralazine reduced blood pressure and dramatically lowered vascular morbidity and mortality. A number of subsequent studies confirmed that control of hypertension was necessary to reduce the burden of cardiovascular diseases and stroke.

In large part because of the data from the Framingham study, cholesterol-lowering and antidiabetic drugs also became standard for the prevention and reduction of cardiovascular disease in the 1970s and 80s. Thanks to all of these developments there has been a threefold reduction in mortality due to heart disease and eightfold due to stroke.

There is allure in this analogy. If high blood pressure, high cholesterol, and high glucose have all been demonstrated to eventually cause cardiovascular disease, why should we not accept that high brain amyloid and tau can eventually cause neurodegenerative disease? Just as hypertension lurks before a stroke, amyloidosis precedes dementia.

However, there is a fundamental difference in the Framingham study that none of the studies on Alzheimer's have replicated, which allows hypertension to be elevated to the state of causality it is now recognized with: the Framingham cohort study was free of hypotheses. It did not start by testing the idea that high blood pressure was going to cluster disproportionately in those who would go on to have heart attacks and strokes. In fact, it did not even select people on the basis of their blood pressures in order to achieve a proportion of hypertensive participants. It measured blood pressure prospectively while capturing many other health parameters in thousands of normal individuals and followed them for many years until some developed "events" of interest. It eventually was recognized that many more of those with hypertension at the time of their recruitment went on to develop strokes or heart attacks in greater numbers than those who had normal blood pressures.

Critically, the association between hypertension and strokes and heart attacks was subsequently proven to be causal when placebo-controlled clinical trials of drugs capable of reducing blood pressure showed that lower rates of stroke and heart attacks were more common among those who were in the treated group (and responded to the hypotensive effect of these drugs) compared to those who were in the placebo group.

While it is true that many of those with brain amyloidosis go on to develop dementia, the association between high amounts of amyloid and dementia has never proven to be causal of Alzheimer's disease. As discussed in Chapter 10, of the 32 Phase 2 and 3 clinical trials, not only have all been negative; nearly 40% of these trials have worsened people in the treated group compared to those in the placebo group. In fact, the majority of the therapies tested over the last decade effectively lowered the levels of brain amyloid, as they were designed to do, yet they deteriorated cognition and accelerated brain atrophy.

The analogy is further disrupted by the fact that, unlike the many causes of heart attacks and strokes, which includes hypertension, hypercholesterolemia, and diabetes, we assume the whole of Alzheimer's is ultimately due to the unifying "toxic" effect of high amyloid and tau. While the several causes of cardiovascular disease are weighted separately and approached on a per-patient basis, no such personalized approach to treatment exists for people with a diagnosis of Alzheimer's disease.

Led by Clifford Jack, a group of experts working on behalf of the National Institute on Aging–Alzheimer Association (NIA-AA) proposed the so-called A/T/N research framework for the diagnosis of Alzheimer's disease throughout the entire set of known possibilities with regards to amyloid, tau, and loss of neurons.[157] According to this research framework, abnormal amyloid but normal tau biomarker (A+T–) denotes "Alzheimer pathologic change," but both amyloid and tau (A+T+) are required for the diagnosis of Alzheimer's disease, even in the absence of brain degeneration (A+T+N–). Neurodegeneration is conceived as the most severe Alzheimer's stage since it implies the death of neurons in at least some regions of the brain, and can co-occur with (A+T+N+) or without amyloid or tau (A–T–N+). The *Alzheimer disease spectrum*, also referred to as *Alzheimer continuum* became the umbrella term for any A+ individual, healthy or impaired, in whom tau could be normal, abnormal, or unknown.

As we noted earlier, the A/T/N framework created a "misalignment" between the established symptoms we have come to accept in order for Alzheimer's disease to be clinically defined and the biomarker-based definition. And this is the relevant question that pertains to such redefinition: is a normal 60-year-old person discovered to be in the A+ of the *Alzheimer continuum* the perfect candidate for trials to pre-empt dementia in the future?

If biomarker-defined Alzheimer's disease is a way to mark clinically defined Alzheimer's disease before it becomes apparent, then the answer is Yes.

Graphing such a relationship would look like what is depicted below: A+ is detectable many years before the symptoms of dementia appear. If we assume the theoretical prevalence of A+ in the population is 30% around the age of 60 years, and A+ precedes dementia by at least 10 years, the prevalence of Alzheimer's dementia in this group would reach at least 20% by the age of 70, and about 30% by the age of 80. Also, if A+ predicts dementia within a lifetime, nearly 100% of A+ people will become demented before the age of 85. If the prevalence of A+ is around 60% by age of 85, the prevalence of dementia should be theoretically close to 60%.

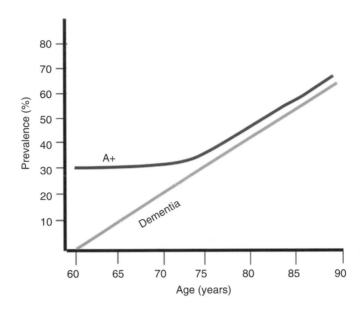

What is the actual lifetime prevalence of A+ and dementia in the population?

To answer this question, Cliff Jack and his colleagues used data from a population-based cohort of 5,213 individuals participating in three studies belonging to the Mayo Clinic Study of Aging from Olmsted County, Minnesota.[158] Positron emission tomography was used to scan brains for amyloid (using Pittsburgh Compound B) and tau (flortaucipir). The ages of the participants were from 60 to 89 years.

The results were quite different to what would have been expected of a biomarker predicting dementia accurately because it is the one that defines it.

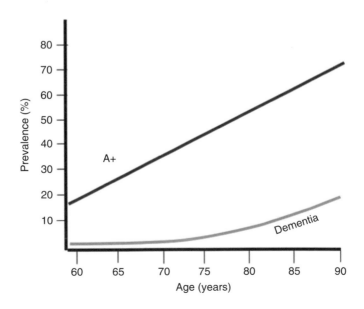

Notice that the prevalence of A+ goes from around 15% at age 60 to 70% by age 90. Conversely, the prevalence of Alzheimer's dementia hovered in the single digits until about age 85, when it reaches 10%. The prevalence of dementia never reaches 20% even at the age of 90. Not only do these curves never meet but in fact they diverge until about the age of 85, when they seem to begin running in parallel. After that, amyloid and dementia seem to increase roughly linearly.

The actual lifetime prevalence of 85-year-old A+ people without dementia is *six times* greater (10% vs. 60%) than that of clinically defined Alzheimer's dementia. Put explicitly, most people with high brain amyloid will never develop Alzheimer's disease. In fact, for the largest chunk of a normal lifetime the prevalence of A+ and dementia separate rather than come together.

Should we trust a test of a disease that is associated with greater likelihood of not developing such disease over a normal life span?

This is the major conclusion by the authors: "… Most patients with biologically defined Alzheimer disease are not symptomatic, which creates potential confusion around the definition of Alzheimer disease."

It is indeed confusing. If our amyloid-begets-Alzheimer's narrative is the one to prevail, should we inform everyone in the A+ spectrum that they should know they have Alzheimer's even if they will never develop the dementia it supposedly predicts?

If beta-amyloid defines Alzheimer's disease, the reliance on this as a marker of disease is creating an artificially inflated prevalence of Alzheimer's dementia, one that never materializes during life. Should this data inform public health planners and public and private health agencies on the future epidemic of Alzheimer's disease? It is hard to see how. And we would offer a "No" to the question we posed earlier of whether a normal 60-year-old person classified within the amyloid spectrum should participate in any antiamyloid trials to minimize the risk of evolving into Alzheimer's dementia.

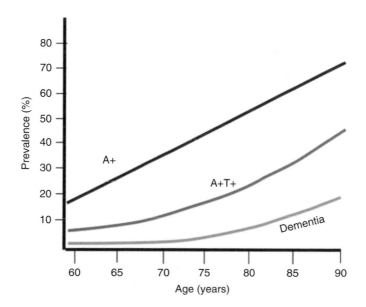

Even if the full biologically defined Alzheimer's disease, that is A+T+, is tested, we are still seeing a large gap. By age 90, "biological Alzheimer's" just reaches 40%, whereas clinically recognizable Alzheimer's disease remains below 20%. The actual lifetime prevalence of 85-year-olds to have biomarker-defined Alzheimer's disease without actual dementia is *three times* greater (10% vs. 30%) than having dementia recognized clinically as Alzheimer's disease.

The authors suggest this finding is not surprising because "in any other disease such as in cancer or diabetes tests can detect disease in both symptomatic and asymptomatic individuals." They put their results in practical terms: "Even though there are no therapies proven to alter clinical outcomes, our data illustrate that a significant opportunity exists to influence public health by intervention in the preclinical phase of the disease if that proves to be efficacious."

Is the "significant opportunity" the one posed by a future antiamyloid treatment "if that proves to be efficacious" to be delivered to normal people in the A+T− or A+T+ *Alzheimer continuum*, considered "preclinical,"[1] with the expectation that fewer will develop dementia?

If there ever is an antiamyloid agent that defies the evidence reviewed in this book and proves to be efficacious (as mentioned in the last chapter, Biogen believes aducanumab may be the last hope in what otherwise has been a string of antiamyloid failures) how might such a significant opportunity be harnessed?

Let's say we would recruit neurologically normal 65-year-old individuals with an A+T− biomarker profile. The rationale of avoiding an A+T+ cohort is twofold: first, according to the amyloid hypothesis, A+T+ individuals are considered more advanced than A+T− since beta-amyloid presumably precipitates the misfolding of tau; second, we would have to design an antiamyloid plus antitau dual-therapy clinical trial, far more complex than a single-therapy antiamyloid trial.

Now let's imagine two scenarios. One in which the amyloid hypothesis of pathogenicity stands despite the many bruises we have highlighted. The other in which most individuals with lots of amyloid are "resistant" to developing dementia; let's say with a ratio of about six A+T− people to one person with dementia of Alzheimer's type (I trust this does not seem farfetched by now).

In the first scenario, half the cohort of 65-year-old A+T− individuals are allocated to an anti-Aβ treatment, the other half to placebo. A minimum period of five years would have to elapse before reviewing the extent to which the rate at which dementia occurs is lower than expected in those on the anti-Aβ treatment than in those on placebo. Using the data from Cliff Jack and colleagues, although we would be hoping for detecting a change within a five-year period, the base rate of dementia is so low to begin with that by the end of the trial, there would likely have been no separation between the groups in terms of dementia prevalence. If the hypothesis that lowering amyloid lowers the prevalence of dementia is correct, the cohort will need to be

---

[1] Normal individuals with biomarkers classifying them as A+T− and A+T+ are considered by the NIA-AA criteria as being in the "preclinical phase." The data reviewed here suggests that most will never become "clinical" (i.e., develop Alzheimer's dementia) and were never, therefore, truly preclinical.

followed for at least 15 years for a difference to start to emerge! This very long window of observation is prohibitively expensive for any funding agency of such clinical trial. Because of cost and logistical feasibility, most clinical trials last between one and three years, a period with little chance of yielding differences in people so resistant to dementia over so many years, despite the "toxicity" of A+.

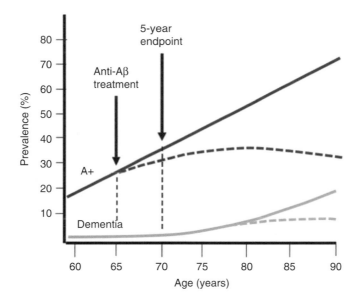

For a protein conceived as toxic, it is remarkable that amyloid can be documented in as many as 30% of everyone by the age of 65 and one of every two 80-year-old individuals. As we have noted from the figure, the prevalence of Alzheimer's dementia does not start to tick up in earnest until at least a decade later, with a slope not matching that of A+ until about the age of 85. Hence, if there is a direct toxic effect from amyloid leading to dementia, such effect is very slow, requiring a span of about two decades to "sync."

Let's move on to the second scenario. As we have reviewed from the oldest-old data, it seems as or more likely that amyloid is a compensatory strategy. This would better explain the divergence between the A+ and dementia curves over the first decade shown in the graph. The prevalence of dementia remains in the low single digits until about 75 years despite a linearly increasing prevalence of A+.

Under this scenario, the pharmacologic removal of amyloid may in fact be counterproductive. As the figure on the next page illustrates, the prevalence of dementia would actually increase because the protective effect afforded by amyloid becomes smaller. However, unlike the situation in the first scenario, it is more likely that a deleterious effect may be captured within the five-year window of a long trial in the treated group compared to the placebo group.

Neither scenario seems particularly attractive for interventions in the preclinical phase of the disease. Nevertheless, amyloid is literally at the center of the dementia universe, a key narrative created by neuroscientists. If this seems confusing, it is because it is. Most people with brain amyloid will never develop dementia.

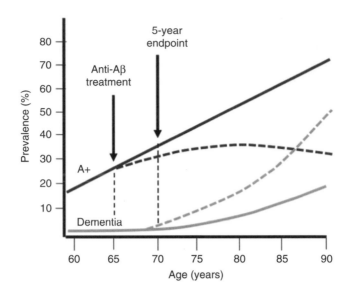

The convergent role of amyloid and tau as the center of the neurological universe is the narrative espoused from most academic corners. It is reminiscent of the same reductionist narrative that made sense when the Earth was known as the center of the universe, under the Ptolemaic system (Figures 29 and 30 in the next two pages). This geocentric model stood for millennia, backed by the observation that the sun and stars spun in circles around us. It was not until Nicolaus Copernicus developed the tools to investigate beyond what the naked eye could see that in 1543 he postulated the Earth may be just another planet in a system with the sun as its center, hurtling through the cosmos. The transition from Ptolemaic geocentrism to Copernican heliocentrism changed the story of our existence and opened the doors to the Scientific Revolution that forever reshaped the ability of humanity to understand and manipulate the world we live in.

We neurologists still rely on the universe we can see. What we observe under the lenses of our microscopes at the time of autopsy remains the compass by which we give reason and order to the symptoms we note in our patients.

While patients see the narrative of diversity in their symptoms, doctors see the narrative of unification in autopsy samples from patients. All the diversity of symptoms ultimately revolve around the "gravitational forces" of the narrative built around amyloid and tau.

We need the same revolution in neurodegenerative diseases as the hypothesis-free Framingham study did for cardiovascular diseases. It is critical to learn how we age into one of the many ways we currently define as Alzheimer's – without assuming "Alzheimer's disease" is the truth we need biological proof for. Amyloid, tau, and alpha-synuclein, among others, may be but satellites in the vast galaxy of our biology (Figure 31). Our "moonshot" is to recognize and distinguish the moon from the Earth and from the Sun – and every element giving life and bringing death around these cosmic bodies of aging.

To the promise and challenges of the "moonshot" we will turn our attention in the next two chapters.

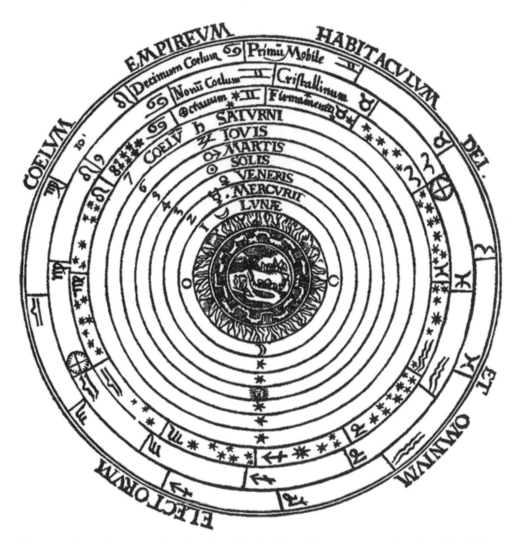

Figure 29 Ptolemaic geocentrism. Formulated by the Alexandrian astronomer and mathematician Ptolemy around AD 150, the geocentric cosmology assumed that the Earth was stationary and at the center of the universe. All heavenly bodies (Sun, Moon, planets, and stars) must travel in uniform motion along the most "perfect" path possible, a circle. The Ptolemaic system persisted until the Copernican system and Kepler's laws of planetary motion displaced the Earth from the center of the universe. (Engraving from Peter Apian's Cosmographia; Antwerp, 1539; copyright in the public domain).

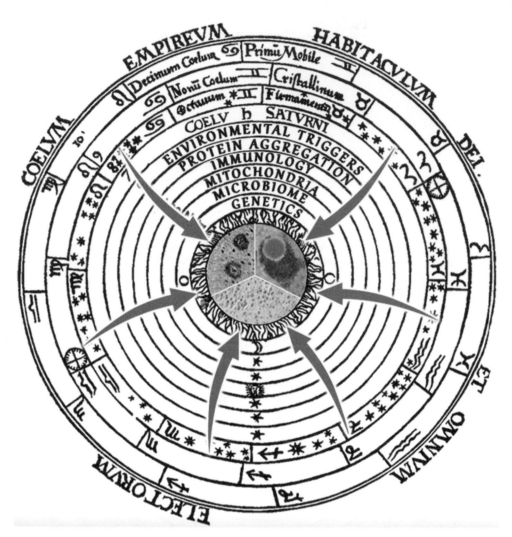

Figure 30 "Tau-lemaic" protein-centrism. The discovery of proteinaceous materials at autopsy has provided a "definitive diagnosis" to all neurodegenerative disorders. According to this cosmology, aggregated proteins such as tau, amyloid, synuclein, and others, are the gravitational forces directing all biological planets into destructive orbits. Such *Tau-lemaic* model has persisted for over a century and has motivated most of the antiaggregation missiles launched over the last two decades – most notably the antiamyloid arsenal, which continues to grow. A new stock pile of antisynuclein ammunition is being widely deployed. (Adaptation of the Cosmographia by Marcia Hartsock).

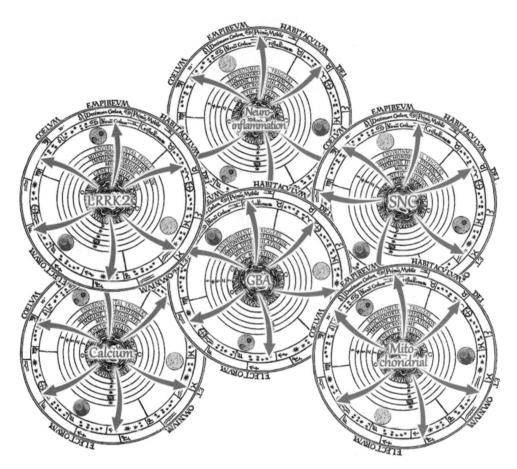

Figure 31 Systems biology revolution. As with the replacement of the Earth-centered universe, prompted by Nicolaus Copernicus and Newton, we are on the brink of the intellectual breakthrough that will bring a veritable Scientific Revolution to the approach to modify neurodegenerative disorders. According to the emerging cosmology, aggregated proteins such as tau, amyloid, synuclein, and others, are but satellites to the greater gravitational forces of biological planets, orbiting around them but only slightly modifying their rotational movements. The systems-biology galaxy will bring an end to the antiaggregation warfare, replacing it with smart combat and precise exit strategies. (Additional adaptation of the Cosmographia by Marcia Hartsock).

Commentary – One Giant Clump

You were born a winner, a warrior, one who defied the odds by surviving the most gruesome battle of them all – the race to the egg. And now that you are a giant, why do you even doubt victory against smaller numbers and wider margins? The only walls that exist are those you have placed in your mind. And whatever obstacles you conceive, exist only because you have forgotten what you have already achieved.

Suzy Kassem, Rise Up and Salute the Sun: The Writings of Suzy Kassem

In June of 2019 I gave a talk to the resident neurologists at the University of Toronto. The talk was titled "Breaking Barriers in Neurodegeneration," in which I gave a summary of what I think are the biggest problems that the Parkinson's disease field faces and some of the things that need to be done to solve them.

We had a great discussion afterwards in which it quickly became clear that almost none of the problems I outlined are unique to the Parkinson's disease field. Here are some of those key issues:

- We don't understand the biology driving these diseases.
- We have been chasing the wrong targets all along.
- Each disease is poorly defined and likely represents a spectrum of many biological disorders.
- There are very few incentives in place to promote the kind of broad collaborative efforts needed to push research forward.
- Science is primarily driven by what publishers and grant reviewers want. This perpetuates a scientific culture that revolves around accepted concepts without prioritizing the needs of society.
- None of our animal models could come close to recapitulating a disease that comes in so many forms.
- Drug development is painfully slow. Even if a cure were discovered in the lab today, it would take 12 to 18 years to get the therapy to patients.
- Patients have inadequate access to the care they need.

So, since almost all of the problems faced are common across disease boundaries, it seems to make sense to break down the divisions separating disease fields and see if we can't achieve more together.

However, this seems to run counter to the direction medicine itself is heading. Precision or personalized medicine is a movement away from grouping patients into large disease clusters and toward precision therapies tailored for specific molecular abnormalities in small groups. So, why should we cluster all these diseases together under one giant umbrella term if the goal is to break them up into even smaller bits?

To that I would say that precision medicine only truly becomes precise when we have molecularly (or at least genetically) defined diseases. To get there we will need to make progress in almost all of the areas mentioned above. Until we have those unique signatures that allow us to properly categorize diseases we need to be disease agnostic and focus on a more general understanding of how biology changes as we age and what are the influences of genetic variants and environmental exposures. In addition, the tools and techniques developed to get us a better understanding of biology and disease cut across classically defined disease boundaries.

This raises the question of whether it makes sense to have laboratories devoted to just Parkinson's or just dementia. Biology does not have an equivalent for what we call Parkinson's or Alzheimer's. Neither is there one for multiple sclerosis, multiple system atrophy, frontotemporal dementia, or progressive supranuclear palsy. All of them are labels that neurologists created to make sense of a spectrum of clinical observations from different patterns of accelerated brain aging.

Our clinical definitions help triage people into groups. For instance, mobility problems are classified as Parkinson's, cognitive impairment as Alzheimer's. However the line separating the two is porous. Most people diagnosed with Parkinson's will experience cognitive decline, and most with Alzheimer's will have their mobility impaired. On autopsy, the amyloid and tau protein buildups we have come to recognize as the hallmarks of the Alzheimer's brain are commonly found in the brains of people with Parkinson's. Conversely, the aggregates of synuclein believed to be responsible for Parkinson's also show up in the brains of people diagnosed with Alzheimer's.

The time to rethink disorders of brain aging has come. Perhaps the most prudent thing to do now is to go back to the drawing board so we can identify, at a molecular level, the unique signatures that correspond with particular expressions of disease states. Only then will we be able to develop the precision therapies needed to effectively combat the growing storm of the aging brain.

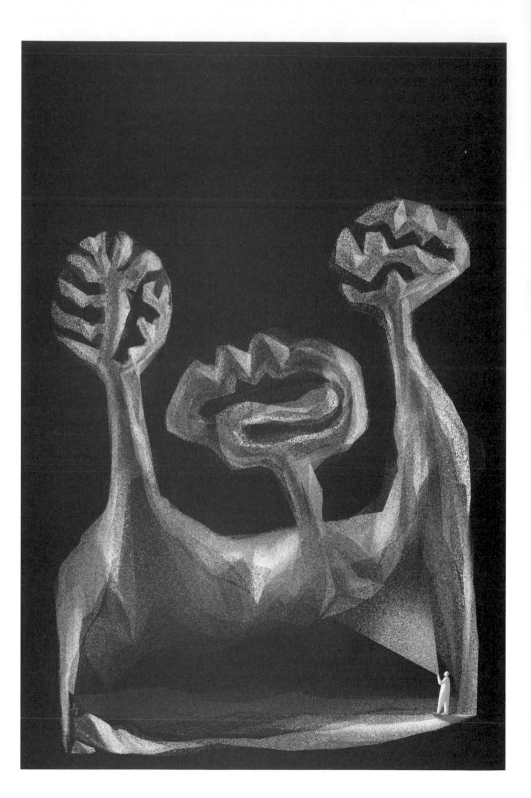

Challenges Viewed from Afar

13

Science is often described as an iterative and cumulative process, a puzzle solved piece by piece, with each piece contributing a few hazy pixels of a much larger picture. But the arrival of a truly powerful new theory in science often feels far from iterative. Rather than explain one observation or phenomenon in a single, pixelated step, an entire field of observations suddenly seems to crystallize into a perfect whole. The effect is almost like watching a puzzle solve itself.

Siddhartha Mukherjee, The Emperor of All Maladies

Marcelo Kauffman, a brilliant neurogeneticist from Buenos Aires, sent me on December 21, 2018 a web link to alert me of an essay by Kevin Mitchell, an associate professor of genetics and neuroscience at Trinity College Dublin, in Ireland. It attempted to provide an editorial perspective on a series of articles recently published on the genomics of psychiatric disorders. Mitchell, the author of *Innate: How the Wiring of Our Brain Shapes Who We Are* (Princeton University Press), writes the *Wiring the Brain* blog, from which his essay was extracted. Kauffman introduced his essay to me by noting, "Surely, some of his arguments will ring true about the reductionist fallacies on which you have focused."

I read the essay as if I was seeing a reflection of our own challenges, from someone else's experience. The concluding paragraphs, copied here, were very telling:

Simply put, nothing really definitive comes out. In fact, the strongest result from these studies is a general one, and it is "negative": there are no convergent patterns of gene expression in adult brain that characterise these various psychiatric conditions.

(…)

Now, defenders of this approach might counter by saying that the first tranche of papers simply present this huge dataset that can now be analysed by many others and that can generate new hypotheses for further study. And there is no doubt that they will generate many more papers.

But it is not clear to me that they actually do generate new hypotheses – not ones that are experimentally testable at any rate. The problem relates to concentrating on the common variant, polygenic component of risk. This involves so many variants, each with such a minuscule effect, that it is almost impossible to follow up on in experimental systems.

I guess if all you have is a hammer, everything looks like a nail. But ultimately, these psychiatric disorders are not a problem genomics alone can solve. At some stage we have to hand the problem over to neuroscientists. This means giving them something they can work with experimentally – not just lists of genes compared to other lists of genes.

My own bet is on rare mutations with large effects, where it may be much more feasible to identify strong biological effects and follow the trajectory of events that leads from altered development or function of some particular cell types and circuits in the developing brain to the ultimate emergence of particular pathophysiological states. (Not that that approach doesn't have its own challenges!)

Mitchell also released a thought-provoking eight-minute lecture on "Irritable Brain Syndrome," which is searchable on YouTube.

Kevin Mitchell's essay read very much like the "reconstruction" part of an international symposium on "Revision vs. Reconstruction" that I and colleagues organized in April 2019. That the field of psychiatry has found itself on a similar revision-vs.-reconstruction dilemma suggested something bigger than us was brewing in neurosciences.

I shared this with Tony Lang, lifelong mentor and also the chair of the "revision vs. reconstruction" meeting. He found the arguments interesting and cogent. He predicted that if we share this information with our faculty, they will argue that a major difference between Parkinson's disease and the psychiatric diseases discussed here is "the clear neuropathological substrate for the majority of cases of Parkinson's and the relationship between the known pathogenic protein and certain genetic forms." He was identifying one near mortal problem for the ushering of the conceptual breakthrough we are advocating: our colleagues' perception that neurology is far ahead of the psychiatric field. That perception exists because while we can boast of the same clinical diversity as psychiatric disorders, we have "considerably more solid grounding in understanding the biological basis for the clinical features of Parkinson's" than, say, schizophrenia or bipolar disorder.

If we agree that neurology may be more advanced than psychiatry because of well-defined pathological basis, blind adherence to this type of "progress" can also be a powerful intellectual opium holding us back. To the extent that psychiatry does not have a convergent pathology for which to claim allegiance, as we do, those working on schizophrenia and bipolar disorder are in fact freer to adopt a model of systems biology divergence while we continue to preach clinico-pathologic convergence.

Dr. Jed Hartings, an associate professor at the University of Cincinnati, has been working on "spreading depolarizations," a phenomena whereby abnormal electrical waves generated after strokes and traumatic brain injuries amplify the original damage. During an email conversation in which I made him aware of neurology's "identity crisis," he wrote back delighted by the parallels he envisioned between our fields. "Reductionism and the 'one disease' viewpoint have dogged these fields [stroke/traumatic brain injury] as well," he wrote. "It seems all of neuroscience is in need of a revolution in order to reset perspective and expectations. I am highly persuaded that there is no single 'cure' for these diseases, and to look for one in clinical trials is the wrong approach… And it starts with better disease classification, or even ditching the idea of classification altogether in favor of the spectrum viewpoint."

He also saw a similarity between his field and ours in terms of the principal explanation for the clinical trial failures discussed earlier: that we are not doing those trials early enough. "This was another nice parallel," he wrote, "along with the flawed idea that we just need to treat earlier (8, 4, 2, 1 hour after stroke/traumatic brain injury) to get the result we want. It's just more of the same approach as focusing on prodromal Parkinson's, with a slight tweak."

The most captivating section of the "Revision vs. Reconstruction" meeting held in April was the "lessons from other fields" section. An audience of neuroscientists listened to a breast cancer and a cystic fibrosis expert. There were several questions for which we were seeking parallelisms. For instance, how many negative trials did it take for them to reject a hypothesis or reconsider an approach to therapy? Did they wrestle with the "once symptoms occur, it may be too late to intervene" argument? Did they go through the process of reconceptualizing a heterogeneous single disease into many biological entities?

You have heard bits and pieces of the breast cancer story. Breast cancer evolved from one disease to many after a randomized clinical trial in 1981 showed that radical mastectomy, which was the only "sensible" treatment at the time, was not superior to quadrantectomy (breast-preserving surgery).[115,118] Breast cancer is now a constellation of pathology–molecular subtypes based on biopsy data but also molecular markers, and multigene expression assays; each of these subtypes exhibit distinct response to treatments, relapse patterns, and long-term survival.[119]

The story of cystic fibrosis is even more poignant because it is a "monogenic" disorder – that is, the disease occurs because *one gene* is mutated; there are no other causes. However, the discovery in 1989 of that gene, *CFTR*,[161] did not move the needle. No treatment was found effective at slowing the disease using the genetic information. Patients could only be managed by clearing fluids from their lungs, until respiratory failure would prove fatal. After the *CFTR* "potentiator" ivacaftor failed in a large trial of patients with cystic fibrosis, it was determined that only the 4% harboring one specific type of *CFTR* mutation (G551D) would respond; none of those with the most common type (Phe508del) could.[162] Subsequently, it took the recruitment of only cystic fibrosis patients with G551D, effectively ruling out 96 of every 100 patients screened, for a promising Phase 2 trial[163] to be turned into a successful Phase 3 trial.[164] The first approval by the US Food and Drug Administration of a disease-modifying intervention for cystic fibrosis occurred 23 years after the discovery of the cystic fibrosis gene, in January of 2012. Although it was effective for only 4% of cystic fibrosis patients, it was of enormous importance. It disproved the ostensibly "clean" one-gene-one-disease concept through the observation that abnormal mutations in the same gene were still giving rise to variations in the expression of the gene in humans that, for the purposes of treatment, represented separate diseases.

Cystic fibrosis is now recognized to be at least seven *classes* of diseases, each with a unique profile of biological changes, even if arising from the same gene. The pool of patients benefiting from disease-modifying treatments has expanded from 4% in 2012 to more than 60% in 2019. This exponential growth was possible because of a focus on molecular (not clinical) subtyping, the development of biomarker platforms that avoided animal models of efficacy, and the synergistic use of multidrug combination of "potentiators" and "correctors" therapies.

If there is a common denominator between the breast cancer and cystic fibrosis stories it is this: the first success was on a small subgroup. There were no yields when breast cancer or cystic fibrosis were unities. Focusing on the modification of small chunks of previously indivisible entities and using the first success to expand the sphere of influence seems a sensible strategy.

"Parkinson's" and "Alzheimer's" are too broad to be tackled. They are, biologically speaking, fictional constructs. The blueprint for conquering these diseases start by studying the many pathways where normal aging can detour into abnormal aging in different individuals – even with the "same disease." We must keep our focus on small but achievable targets, regardless of whether they fall under "Parkinson's," "Alzheimer's", or any other man-made label.

Commentary – The Greatest Story Ever Told

I began to realize that coming in such close contact with my own mortality had changed both nothing and everything. Before my cancer was diagnosed, I knew that someday I would die, but I didn't know when. After the diagnosis, I knew that someday I would die, but I didn't know when. But now I knew it acutely. The problem wasn't really a scientific one. The fact of death is unsettling. Yet there is no other way to live.

Paul Kalanithi, When Breath Becomes Air

Sorry, Jean-Luc Picard, you were wrong, space is not the final frontier, at least not the space up above. No, the final frontier is deep down in the spaces between the cracks in our skin.

I find it a little strange that we know more about the inner workings of stars billions of light years away than we do about the cells that make up who we are. Yet when I close my eyes and picture everything that a cell is and how it came to be, it fills me with far more wonder and awe than anything I see when I turn my head up to the night sky. Oddly enough, I have Parkinson's to thank for that.

It began at the very first lab I visited, run by Dr. Jeanne Loring in San Diego, where I was introduced to one of the great discoveries of modern biology, induced pluripotent stem cells (iPSCs).

Somehow, we figured out how to scrape off a few skin cells, turn those cells back into stem cells, and then direct those stem cells into becoming any cell in our body (Figure 32).

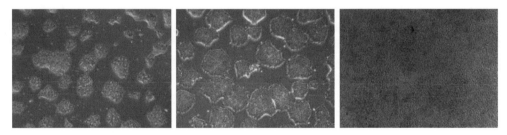

Figure 32 **Human embryonic pluripotent stem cells** being differentiated into dopamine cells at days 2, 4 and 7. Courtesy of Dr. Tilo Kunath's lab at the University of Edinburgh.

The most astounding demonstration of this is the differentiation of stem cells into cardiomyocytes, the muscle cells that make up the heart. At a lab in Toronto I got to see 13-day-old cardiomyocytes under a microscope; cells that not long before were part of a person's skin were now beating in a dish.

Those experiences set me off on a whirlwind of discovery and drove me to learn as much as I could about what else was going on in the biomedical sciences. I went from one lab to another, learning from world experts about the latest in gene editing, immunotherapies, the microbiome, glial cells, neuromodulation, and so much more. It was the ultimate crash course and had me buzzing with anticipation about the future of medicine.

It not only made me more optimistic about the future, it also changed my interpretation of what life and disease are.

To try to explain what I mean, I am going to start with what I think is the greatest story ever told, the story of mitochondria (Figure 33).

First there is the classic tale that all biology students learn ...

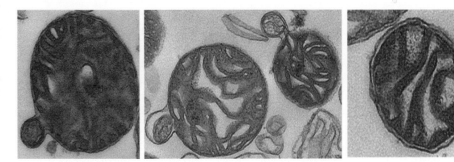

Figure 33 **Pictures of mitochondria**, under electron microscopy. Courtesy of Prof. Heidi McBride's Lab at McGill.

Billions of years ago on Earth, when single-celled organisms ruled the planet, mitochondria floated around independently. They were living things that had their own DNA. A great ancestor of every cell in your body was also floating around at that time. Somehow that cell absorbed a mitochondrion into its structure. Our ancestors' cells found benefit from mitochondria's ability to produce a form of energy called ATP. The mitochondria benefited from the protection it received from its new host. A symbiotic marriage was formed that has allowed life on Earth to thrive and, by extension, humanity to become the dominant species on Earth. You would not be here if that meeting had not happened.

But that is not where the story ends. To fully appreciate mitochondria, you need to take a step inside a dopamine-producing cell.

Our dopamine-producing cells are some of the most robust and intricate pieces of organized matter in the universe. According to David Sulzer, acclaimed neuroscientist at Columbia University, "They are ancient and were first found in an extinct species of worm that is the ancestor to a wide variety of life... One other particularly striking detail of dopamine neurons is they have the longest axons in the body; in mice one dopamine neuron can be half a meter in length, much longer than the mouse itself."

The next astounding piece of this story is just how many mitochondria there are inside each of these neurons. For that I asked Thomas Schwartz, mitochondrial dysfunction expert and professor at Harvard University.

"If you add up all the branches, it is estimated that you would have several meters of axon coming from each (dopamine-producing neuron)," Dr. Schwartz said. "If you take the density of mitochondria in a segment of axon, you can then calculate what the total would be. The number is roughly two million mitochondria in each neuron. That's two million mitochondria frantically consuming oxygen and making ATP, all to keep that one cell alive."

The last piece of this story was told by Heidi McBride, mitochondria fanatic and professor at McGill University. "(Mitochondria) have a hive mentality. This is a big part of trying to figure out why they fuse. When the cell is under stress, the mitochondria band together to protect themselves against being eaten by autophagy or to stop the cell from undergoing apoptosis.[1] When you think about their evolutionary history, it makes sense as

---

[1] Two terms worth defining. Autophagy is a mechanism the cell uses to orderly degrade and recycle cellular components to avoid piling up what is not needed. Apoptosis is a mechanism of programmed self-destruction to dispose of damaged, superfluous, or unwanted cells. Apoptosis gone awry leads to faster aging and death (degeneration); in this scenario, antiapoptotic strategies are desirable.

they used to be bacteria and still have remnants of the original bacteria mechanisms to swarm."

I often rack my brain trying to picture what is happening inside a cell. I think of all the organelles and their known functions and play out in my mind what the world they inhabit might look like. But anything I envision is mostly a creation of my imagination. We do not know enough to fill our mental model of what is going on down there.

———————

It cannot be overstated just how complex our biology is. Each cell in your body has tens of billions of moving parts driven by innumerable chemical reactions that enable each individual cell to communicate, respond to their environment, self-replicate and more. They are the most sophisticated machines in the known universe, and we are made of over 37 trillion of them.

For most of our history we didn't even know they were there. Yet there they were, driving our every thought, feeling and action. Now, finally, we can zoom in and get a bird's-eye view of their worlds to better understand how they do all that they do, and how that impacts all that we do.

The electron microscopy image provided by Prof. Stahlberg (Figure 34) is from a deceased human brain that has been fixed and resin-embedded, then magnified roughly 10,000 times. When alive, every little blob that you see would have been in constant motion, each playing a role in keeping the person alive and healthy.

But from time to time things go wrong. Some blobs break down, others stick to one another forming unhealthy clumps. Yet almost every time our cells figure out how to either fix or contain the problem.

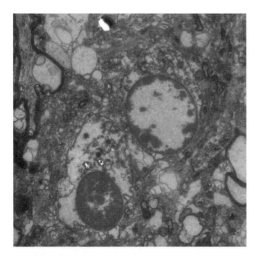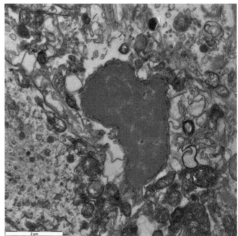

Figure 34 **Electron microscopy images** made available by Prof. Henning Stahlberg and the Stahlberg group at C-CINA, Biozentrum, University of Basel. The image on the left is a cluster of cells inside a deceased human brain magnified roughly 10,000 times. The image on the right is of a dying cell, the process of degeneration can be seen. The nucleus becomes misshapen, the DNA condenses and clumps together and the nuclear membrane is disrupted. The cytoplasm surrounding the nucleus shows many disrupted cellular components such as mitochondria, various vesicles as well as fragmented membranes.

There are rare occasions, however, when damage spirals out of control. In the second image something has gone wrong. The membrane separating the now Africa-shaped nucleus from the rest of the cell is starting to break down as the DNA condenses and clumps together. Before long the disorder will snowball and result in the death of the entire cell.

That is normal, of course. Cells die all the time (which scientists referred to as programmed apoptosis). In the last minute, an estimated 300 million of your cells have died. However, unlike most other cells, the neurons shown above do not get replaced. So as we age their numbers dwindle. In some people that happens faster than in others, and it can cause a variety of motor and non-motor problems. We call that neurodegeneration.

Why this happens and what can be done about it are what researchers studying these diseases are trying to understand. But getting there is as complex a problem as any we know of.

The good news is we are starting to get a handle on the problem thanks in part to new tools that can show us these basic building blocks of biology in unprecedented detail. Powerful electron microscopes now allow us to study our cells and the molecules within them in 3D at a resolution like never before.

But we still have a long way to go before we can even dream of fully understanding what is going on inside us. We may not even be equipped with the language necessary to describe in enough detail something so complicated. Yet we try to make sense of it anyway, which often leaves us rushing to hasty conclusions. We are predisposed to look for order, patterns, and meaning, often seeing them where none exist. We are uncomfortable with uncertainty and get drawn toward simple explanations over complex truths.

It is only natural that when confronted with a challenge as daunting as the biology of neurodegenerative disease that we fall into the trap of confusing evidence for reason.

But we should not despair. While understanding the scale of the problem may make the solution seem out of reach, there is a valuable lesson that an appreciation of the complexity of biology has for us. Simply put, while there are things going wrong inside some of us that make life more challenging than it used to be, there are trillions upon trillions of things going right that make life at all possible.

Life is the greatest story the universe has ever told. At one time it was just a single microscopic blob floating in a primordial ocean somewhere. Now it blankets almost every square inch of Earth and fills each of us with a vast symphony of cells that let us see, touch, hear, smell, and experience the world.

One day, when just enough of our cells die, this experience will end. But instead of getting discouraged by our failures to intervene, we are best served by embracing the complexity and the uncertainty inherent in the challenges life presents. Remember all that must be going right just to be able to confront these challenges in the first place.

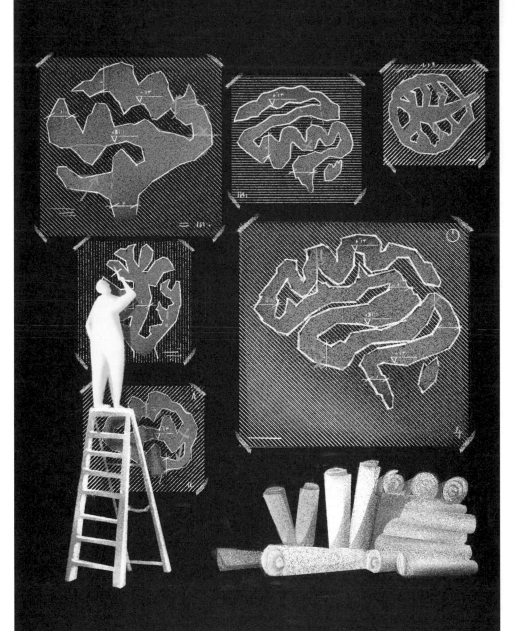

Chapter 14

The Moonshot: Population-Based Studies of Aging

Here is one way to conceptualize NASA's heroic era: in 1961, Kennedy gave his "moon speech" to Congress, charging them to put an American on the moon "before the decade is out." In the eight years that unspooled between Kennedy's speech and Neil Armstrong's first historic bootprint, NASA, a newborn government agency, established sites and campuses in Texas, Florida, Alabama, California, Ohio, Maryland, Mississippi, Virginia, and the District of Columbia; awarded multi-million-dollar contracts and hired four hundred thousand workers; built a fully functioning moon port in a formerly uninhabited swamp; designed and constructed a moonfaring rocket, spacecraft, lunar lander, and space suits; sent astronauts repeatedly into orbit, where they ventured out of their spacecraft on umbilical tethers and practiced rendezvous techniques; sent astronauts to orbit the moon, where they mapped out the best landing sites; all culminating in the final, triumphant moment when they sent Neil Armstrong and Buzz Aldrin to step out of their lunar module and bounce about on the moon, perfectly safe within their space suits. All of this, start to finish, was accomplished in those eight years.

Margaret Lazarus Dean, Leaving Orbit: Notes from the Last Days of American Spaceflight

Throughout this book there has been one theme permeating each chapter: Parkinson's and Alzheimer's are not two distinct diseases but a spectrum of disorders. The stories created for each are as compelling as they are fictitious. There is no such thing as Parkinson's disease. There is no such thing as Alzheimer's disease. These are but powerful ideas.

The time has come to accept that any mechanistic discoveries related to a form of Parkinson's, especially the genetic ones, such as those due to *GBA* mutations, are potential targets for therapeutic development for only those subtypes. No treatment revolving around one mechanistic discovery can be expected to slow the progression of diseases as complex and multifaceted as Parkinson's or Alzheimer's, let alone "cure" them.

We know we will have begun the application of this conceptual breakthrough when we are ready to accept that the first success in disease-modifying treatments will only apply to a small Parkinson's or Alzheimer's subpopulation targeted. This small group will be unique from others in its suitability to respond to the treatment under investigation.

To get there we will first need a paradigm shift in our hunt for biomarkers.

The major change in biomarker development is also the most difficult. Rather than studying the biological abnormalities of people we have definitions for (such as "Parkinson's disease" or "Alzheimer's disease," defined by a neurological evaluation at the bedside) we should study aging first. Instead of continuing to assemble large "Parkinson's disease" cohorts, we should study people aging with a wide range of neurodegenerative disorders.

The questions we are currently asking are a variation of these:

"What is different about the people with tremor versus those who do not have tremor?" "What marker distinguishes a group of cognitively impaired people from a group we define as cognitively preserved?"

But the question needs to be asked in reverse of what is natural (Figure 35):

"Who are those in the population with an abnormality in the range of [X signal] that can be targetable by [X intervention] to normalize such biological change and prevent or attenuate the expression of disease?"

With very large populations, in the thousands rather than hundreds, we will have the statistical power to reverse the question currently asked in ongoing biomarker-discovery cohorts.

This change requires embracing the principle that a bedside diagnosis does not represent a biological truth. Therefore, clinical definitions should not anchor the analyses. Instead, biological outliers dictate what biological subtypes of disease exist. Regardless of how clinically diverse these subgroups may still be, their molecular homogeneity render them potentially targetable for molecular interventions that may already exist (for a glimpse, many in the "graveyard" shown in Chapter 8 can be resuscitated if appropriate candidates are found).

Only future population-based studies of aging applying analytic approaches to biospecimens of large cohorts of aging people anchored on biological signals instead of clinical

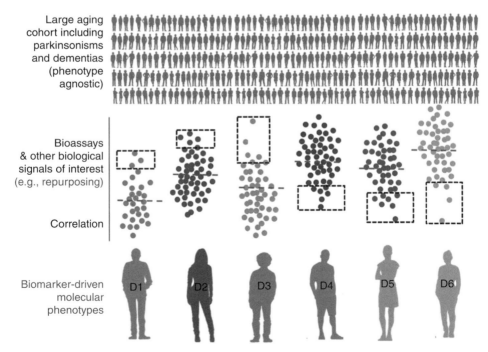

Figure 35 Ideal disease subtyping strategy. The generation of disease subtypes would ideally be "agnostic" to phenotype or clinical diagnosis. In this case, the "gold standard" for subtyping people are the signals of biologic interest. These would generate smaller but more molecularly homogeneous subtypes, suitable for specific therapeutic targeting.

diagnoses will yield molecularly targetable subsets of patients with neurodegenerative diseases.

In other words, we need to remove all preconceived notions and inherent biases, and study diseases of brain aging as agnostically as possible.

As of May 1, 2019, at the University of Cincinnati, we launched such a population-based study aiming to recruit 5,000 people; 4,000 of whom will have a diverse range of neurodegenerative disorders. With the understanding that we don't know where Parkinson's ends and Alzheimer's begins, biologically speaking, the entry criteria for the Cincinnati Cohort Biomarker Program (CCBP) is deliberately inclusive. We are recruiting patients with Parkinson's disease and related parkinsonisms (e.g., progressive supranuclear palsy, multiple system atrophy, corticobasal syndrome, etc.) as well as Alzheimer's and other dementias (e.g., dementia with Lewy bodies, frontotemporal dementias, primary progressive aphasias, etc.). The study has been funded through philanthropy, with major investment by the James J. and Joan A. Gardner Family Foundation as well as intellectual investment from several colleagues from the Parkinson Study Group, the largest not-for-profit scientific network of Parkinson centers in North America. We expect the findings from this long and labor-intensive study will shed light on the many molecular causes of late-onset neurodegenerative disease and to advance us into the era of neuroprotective therapies – and the first cure before the end of the 2020s.

Commentary – The Bet

Being mortal is about the struggle to cope with the constraints of our biology, with the limits set by genes and cells and flesh and bone. Medical science has given us remarkable power to push against these limits, and the potential value of this power was a central reason I became a doctor. But again and again, I have seen the damage we in medicine do when we fail to acknowledge that such power is finite and always will be. We've been wrong about what our job is in medicine. We think our job is to ensure health and survival. But really it is larger than that. It is to enable well-being. And well-being is about the reasons one wishes to be alive. Those reasons matter not just at the end of life, or when debility comes, but all along the way. Whenever serious sickness or injury strikes and your body or mind breaks down, the vital questions are the same: What is your understanding of the situation and its potential outcomes? What are your fears and what are your hopes? What are the trade-offs you are willing to make and not willing to make? And what is the course of action that best serves this understanding?

Atul Gawande, Being Mortal: Medicine and What Matters in the End

The changes outlined in the chapters above, while necessary, are unlikely to be adopted quickly. Reform takes time. Which leads to one rather unsettling conclusion: medical science will not have a solution to these diseases ready within a timeframe relevant to most who are already diagnosed.

And, if that wasn't bad enough, the prevalence of these diseases is growing quickly, the number of people expected to be diagnosed with Parkinson's alone is set to double over the next 20 years.[165]

So, what are patients to do while we wait for the field to sort itself out? How can we keep ourselves healthy enough to actually be able to benefit from any disease-modifying therapy of the future?

Along the way I have met a handful of patients described dismissively by some neurologists as "outliers." These are individuals who managed to significantly reverse their symptoms or at least halt progression. The common theme among these individuals is simple: diet and exercise, taken not in moderation, but to the extreme.

This is not exactly earth-shattering news. Exercise and a healthy lifestyle have long been known to be associated with better outcomes for people with Parkinson's. But what is the optimal "dose?" How much ramping up of exercise is needed to get the most benefit? What kind of exercise is best? Which foods should people be eating? Which should they avoid?

Unfortunately, the studies have not been done. They are difficult to do, and there isn't exactly the same kind of incentive for doing trials on exercise as there are for a drug that could be put on pharmacy shelves.

But we can still look to those outliers for lessons. One such individual is Dr. Karen Raphael, clinical scientist at NYU and a person living with Parkinson's. During an interview I asked her to describe her story.

I need to start by saying that I am a case study. As a research scientist, I'd say that an individual's experience offers a tool for hypothesis generation, but itself is not proof of anything.

I was diagnosed about eight years ago. The first thing I do whenever I have a question about virtually anything is look to the primary research literature. At that time, research in neuroprotective strategies pointed to the idea of rodents running on a treadmill for a very long time having some effect on neuroplasticity, so I started with that. Then I found a movement disorder specialist who said to me that, "There is no such thing as too much exercise for a person with PD". That doctor, like myself, is very involved in clinical research, so she understood the cognitive and physical demands that my job placed on me. When I met her I had three years left on a grant from the NIH, and she told me that, given my symptoms at the time, I should expect that to be my last grant. But, here I am, eight years later, really doing quite well and still getting funded.

I had never been an athlete, but I am relatively assertive, and from college until today (I'm now 63), I have always been physically active. I actually had my first clear symptom when I froze (a common mid-stage symptom of the disease) on a trek to Everest base camp. So, I was already fit. It was probably less difficult for me than it might be for some others to step it up to the next level of fitness. However, when I was diagnosed at 55, my PD was probably more advanced than most who first get diagnosed. I had to take far more than the normal amount of levodopa to get myself back to an acceptable level. Once it was clear what was happening to me, my family and I moved to a building with an elevator to prepare for the possibility that I was not going to be ambulatory for much longer. We also made sure the building had a gym so I could get up at 4:30 a.m. and exercise after walking my dogs.

After about two years of exercising every single day, which included at least 90 minutes of running on a treadmill at a pretty intense pace, I started noticing a decrease in my "off" periods. With the blessing of my neurologist, I reduced the amount of levodopa I was taking. Now, another 18 months later, I don't get off periods anymore. Even if I skip a dose or two, I am okay, and I no longer have any tremor or rigidity.

I have heard several stories similar to Karen's along the way. But, as she mentioned, these individual stories are proof of nothing, though told collectively they start to leave a trail of breadcrumbs.

Another source of these breadcrumbs for me has been the European Parkinson's Therapy Center in Northern Italy. On two separate occasions I have spent two weeks at the foot of the Italian Alps receiving intensive daily physiotherapy specially designed for the movement abnormalities associated with Parkinson's disease.

The center was built by Alex Reed, an Englishman who moved to Italy for work in his 30s, stayed, got married, had kids, and was living the good life until he was diagnosed with Parkinson's disease. He soon realized that what was needed were dedicated neurotherapy centers where people with Parkinson's could go to receive the personalized care they need to properly manage their condition.

Each time I have gone I have seen the marked improvements patients can make in just a couple weeks of intensive therapy. Men and women who came limping in on canes left able to walk unassisted, others who could barely get up from their chairs felt confident enough by the end to get in taxis by themselves.

I bet that a network of these centers designed to optimize everything we know about brain health and apply the lessons learned from all the outliers out there would help more people than any of the disease-modifying therapies currently in development.

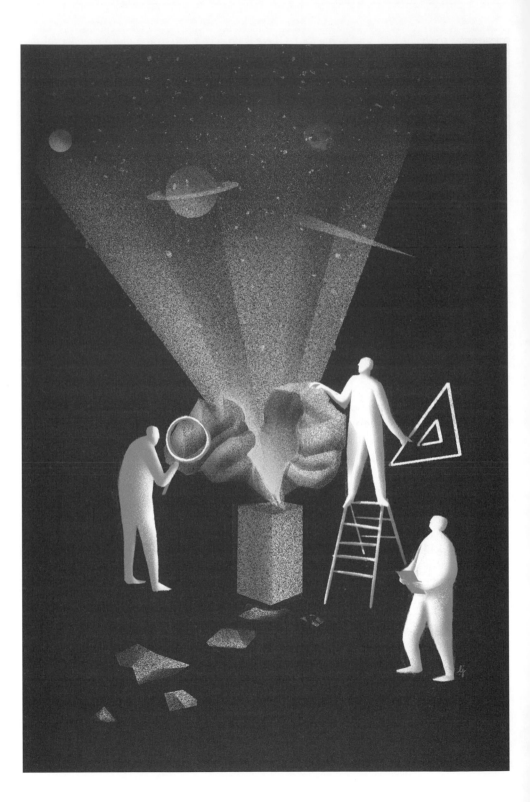

Chapter 15

Predictions for the 2020s and Beyond

This chapter was adapted from Espay and Lang, "Parkinson diseases in the 2020s and Beyond: Replacing Clinico-Pathologic Convergence with Systems Biology Divergence." *J Parkinsons Dis* 2018;8(s1):S59–S64. The article was published in a special edition of the Journal of Parkinson's Disease dedicated to predicting the direction of the next 20 years of research.

Like other fields of medicine, neurodegenerative disorders will move from reductionism, in which any evidence about aspects of a disease inform a global disease, to systems biology, in which genetic and biological signals prevail as anchors for how diseases are subtyped, diagnosed and treated. The recognition that the manner in which a disease expresses does not predict an underlying biology will allow us to move to a biology-first approach to studying diseases of brain aging.

Many concepts providing the relief of convergence (*reductionism*, explaining a range of phenomena as belonging together in order to make sense of the world) will have to be replaced by the anxiety of divergence (no single explanation can sum the range of all observations).

These are the predictions for the 2020s and Beyond (Table 7):

Prediction 1. No longer one puzzle, but many. Parkinson's will cease to represent a combination of many cellular abnormalities that confluence into a single complex "puzzle." In the early 2020s, we will witness the first therapeutic success in a cohort of genetic Parkinson's disease (probably in those with *GBA* mutations). This will be followed by another failure as the new "anti-GBA" therapy is next tested in a cohort of sporadic (*non-GBA*-mutated) Parkinson's disease, even if selected on the basis of an enzymatic marker such as low glucocerebrosidase. The field will finally assess this negative outcome as the final evidence that GBA-associated Parkinson's disease is a distinct disease and not a piece in the "Parkinson Puzzle." A substantial cohort of researchers will still advocate for a repeat trial with "prodromal" (prediagnosis) patients. By 2025, we will no longer assume that therapies that might work for any disease subtype might work for everyone with sporadic Parkinson's disease. Extensive efforts will be undertaken to construct separate diagnostic criteria that incorporate clinical as well as genetic, molecular and pathologic biomarkers for each Parkinson's subtype.

Prediction 2. Biomarker-based selection of patients for trials. Animal models will be used to confirm human disease-based hypotheses, not to create new ones. Animal models will no longer be relied upon to "recapitulate the complexity of a human disease" but to understand specific mechanisms suggested by studies on biospecimens and neuroimaging

Table 7 Reductionism and related ideas that will die

Idea	Why it makes sense	Why it will die
Unification	Few principles must explain many natural phenomena. Mathematics can explain natural patterns.	Mathematics isn't physics. We can only construct approximate models.*
Essentialism	People and events must belong to discrete categories.	There exists a continuous spectrum of intermediates.
Cause–Effect	Events must be organized into chains of causes and effects. A gene seems to cause a trait like height or a disease such as cancer.	Complex dynamical systems of living organisms have patterns of information flow that defy our tools for storytelling.
Linnaean Classification	The vast biological diversity can be ordered based on the description of their similarities and differences.	Taxonomies do not equate with basic biological processes, impeding discovery of treatments.
One Genome per Individual	Single-cell sequencing technology works because all 37 trillion cells have the same copy of one's genome.	A high proportion of brain cells have structural DNA variants (mosaicism).
Race	Skin color, hair form, cranial shape cluster into some diseases. Racial groups must give order to biology.	Racial patterns are complex genetic mixtures created by the sharing of similar exposures.
Nature versus Nurture	You can separate one from the other like Newtonian space and time: heritability is immutable.	As Einsteinian spacetime, they are intertwined. Heritability is affected by the environment.
Big Data	Larger n is better because we can detect small effects. More events and effects become salient.	Significant effects on low n means effect is bigger. Big data may be 99% irrelevant.

Underlying Constructs	
Reductionism: PD as a clinico-pathologic entity	**Systems Biology: PD as a collection of biological entities**
A complex system is nothing but the sum of its parts and can be reduced to its individual constituents. Exceptions to this model are physiological "noise" obscuring the "true" signal.	"Noise" turns into profiles of unique biological systems or subsystems evolving in humans into intricate phenotypes that cannot be reduced.

Inspired from *This Idea Must Die: Scientific Theories That Are Blocking Progress.*[166]
* Even the most sacred unifications are approximations: equations describing electricity and magnetism are perfectly symmetric only in an empty space.
Unification from Marcelo Gleiser (theoretical physicist); *Essentialism* from Richard Dawkins (evolutionary biologist); *Cause and Effect* from W. Daniel Hillis (physicist); *Linnaean Classification* ("Numbering Nature") from Kurt Gray (social psychologist); *One Genome per Individual* from Eric J. Topol (professor of genomics); *Race* from Nina Jablonski (biological anthropologist); *Nature versus Nurture* from Timo Hannay (director of *Digital Science*); and *Big Data* from Melanie Swan (applied genomics expert).

techniques in *humans*. Potential therapies affecting a presumed disease pathway in an animal model will require a demonstration that the same mechanism is active and causal in the potential recipients to enroll. National Institutes of Health research applications will abolish the requirement that prospective trials in humans should be first reproduced in mice or insist on review policies that enforce animal models as the gold standard for predicting the safety and efficacy of promising drugs. High-risk/high-gain, non-hypothesis-based (exploratory) proposals will begin to replace hypothesis-based proposals.

Prediction 3. Smaller, smarter clinical trials. Future trials will select and stratify study participants by mechanism and not clinical features. These trials will include tens of biologically homogenous subjects (with "homogeneity" defined by molecular/biological abnormalities suitable for a targeted molecular/biological intervention) rather than hundreds of clinically defined early or even "prodromal" patients lacking such biomarker(s). Treatments with putative disease-modifying properties, considered ineffective in prior large clinical trials, will be re-examined as potentially useful for a smaller subset of biologically defined individuals. Traditional phases of clinical trial development (preclinical and clinical phases 1 through 3) will be replaced with nimbler *learning and confirming* phases.[167] Adaptive trial designs will become standard to quickly eliminate futile interventions and replace them with others, as well as to assess the effect of combining more than one treatment in the same cohort. Trials of "cocktail" treatments will harness additional potential benefits by targeting more than one dominant pathogenic mechanism in any given molecular disease subtype.[168]

Prediction 4. Larger, phenotype-agnostic biomarker studies of aging. Large population-based aging cohorts will facilitate analyses anchored on outlying biological signals, especially those reflective of mechanisms for which putative therapies already exist. Biomarker-defined subgroups may still not segregate into homogeneous clinical clusters. Discoveries made on biomarker-driven phenotype-agnostic studies of aging will reinvigorate the efforts on repurposing medications (drugs already developed but considered "futile" by virtue of prior negative clinical trials in non-biomarker-defined populations). Proof-of-concept clinical trials of promising disease-modifying drugs targeting specific causal biological mechanisms will be embedded within biomarker-development cohorts of individuals with biological evidence of the targeted dysfunction.

The decades following 2020 will witness a seismic change in the approach to ushering precision medicine for Parkinson's disease. The "sum of parts" clinico-pathologic reductionism that has defined it as a single but heterogeneous disease will be fully replaced with biomarker development and disease modification efforts responsive to individual combinations of clinical, pathologic, genetic, and molecular/biologic features.

The idea of Parkinson's disease representing many diseases has received ceremonious lip service for most of the past 15 years,[1] but walking the talk will soon begin in earnest. Only an agnostic, non-hypothesis-driven approach to biomarker development, anticipated to be far more expensive than the current phenotype-based biomarker programs, will serve to identify biomarkers of causative pathological mechanisms and distinguish them from non-specific or late mechanisms. Such a diagnostic shift will also engender a therapeutic testing paradigm for neuroprotection, emulating the approach in oncology, using a tailored biology-specific but multiple-mechanism strategy.

The historical development of other fields in medicine has shown that diseases defined by their observable features, such as we currently do for Parkinson's and Alzheimer's diseases, tend to be replaced by several (or many) molecular diseases. A departure from the clinico-pathologic disease model on which Parkinson's and Alzheimer's have been based, and for which protein aggregation continues to stimulate therapeutic endeavors, will also require accepting that the first proven neuroprotective therapy may only work on just 1% or 2% of those currently classified as having "Alzheimer's disease" or "Parkinson's disease."

This first cure, however restricted it may be, will become the first in a string of successes marking the adoption of biomarker-driven disease subtyping for neurodegenerative disorders. It will also introduce the primacy of biology over clinical definitions into neurology. The century of the convergent clinico-pathologic disease model for Parkinson's, Alzheimer's, and other diseases of brain aging will then give rise to the era of a divergent systems-biology approach to biomarker validation and clinical trials of neuroprotective and neurorestorative approaches.

Then, and only then, will the field of neurodegenerative diseases join the rest of medicine.

Commentary – A New Hope

I find your lack of faith disturbing.
Darth Vader

My journey with this disease began in Tikal, Guatemala when I was 25 years old. At the end of a long hike through Mayan ruins, we stopped, perched atop a temple to take in the jungle canopy stretched all around us. It was then that I felt the first signs that something was wrong, a slight twitching of my right foot. It passed quickly, long enough to leave an impression but not long enough to warrant doing anything about it. Not that it mattered. To this day there isn't anything anyone could have done for it. But that won't be true for long.

The general direction of the field of Parkinson's research today can be summed up in two words – Detect and Stop. Find tools or markers that can identify the earliest signs of disease and then develop therapies that can slow or stop it from advancing.

That is the future this book is trying to speed us toward. In that future, at a routine checkup in a doctor's office, an early signature of my disease would have been detected long before that tremor became noticeable. My doctor would then have prescribed a therapy tailored to fit my unique biological makeup, it probably would consist of just a pill or two taken daily, or a simple one-time injection. That would essentially be it, this whole ordeal that is Parkinson's disease would be reduced to a few visits in a doctor's office. If broadly applied, this would pretty much eradicate all future incidents of this disease.

But we aren't there yet. However, there is good reason to be optimistic that that won't be the case for long thanks to some exciting projects going on all around the world.

The Linked Clinical Trials (LCT) Program

LCT is the brainchild of Dr. Richard Wyse, director of research for The Cure Parkinson's Trust (CPT). The story of CPT is itself an incredibly inspiring tale as the charity was co-founded by four people with Parkinson's including the late Tom Isaacs who walked the entire coastline of Britain to raise funds for a cure. The LCT attempts to identify drugs that might have therapeutic use in Parkinson's disease. Many of these are repurposed drugs which show promise because if successful they can significantly reduce the amount of time it takes to get through the arduous clinical trial process.

Recently LCT has embarked on some rather innovative and ambitious projects. Perhaps the grandest of them is the Australian Parkinson's Mission which was recently launched in partnership with the government of Australia where they will soon start the first multidrug treatment trial in Parkinson's. The trial will have five arms testing four different compounds plus one placebo control group. A critical part of this trial is that they will conduct extensive genetic and molecular characterization of trial participants in an attempt to ascertain what specific traits distinguish positive responders of the drugs in question from negative responders.[169] This is an important step forward, many failed trials of the past worked for some individuals in the trial but we were unable to tell who. Hopefully, thanks in part to the LCT, future trials will not make the same mistake.

The Silverstein Foundation

A new force has emerged of late that is reshaping the direction of biomedical research around the globe. That is the entry of venture capital firms into the biotech industry. This new funding paradigm has been largely responsible for an explosion of smaller biotech companies in the neurodegenerative field, as well as an immense growth in the number of active trials.

This influx is also helping bridge the divide between academia and industry, and between startups and big pharma. This is creating a wealth of new opportunities, as illustrated in this excerpt from my interview with Dr. Kalpana Merchant who spent 25 years as an executive in the pharmaceutical industry.

> The other side of the equation is the so-called divide between big pharma and small pharma or biotechs, which is somewhat artificial. Mid- and small-sized companies have come up and filled some of the gap to the point that today we have the largest number of clinical and discovery-stage programs for Parkinson's disease that I have ever seen. More importantly, some of these small companies have the freedom to pursue innovative approaches that target specific, and thereby smaller patient populations, without being encumbered by comparison to other therapeutic areas or larger market size considerations. Although such approaches are not at all beyond the risk of failures, a number of them will likely deliver sufficient clinical stage data to de-risk the approach and make it attractive for big pharma's engagement into the program to conduct larger trials and take it to the market. Since leaving big pharma I have seen many of these smaller companies filling gaps in both earlier discovery and clinical development phase that some large pharma may be walking away from. This new ecosystem is working and as a result PD is one of the areas where venture capital support is actually on the rise.[Oct 28, 2018]

Perhaps the biggest splashes made in 2019 from this new ecosystem has come from The Silverstein Foundation. The founder, Jonathan Silverstein, is a global partner at OrbiMed, one of the largest healthcare-dedicated investment firms in the world. Jonathan himself was diagnosed with Parkinson's in February 2017 and soon afterwards decided to take what he had learned from his decades spent helping OrbiMed grow and apply it to accelerating the development of therapies for Parkinson's. His foundation has one clear goal: pursue and invest in research towards new therapies for the treatment of Parkinson's Disease for GBA mutation carriers.

The company which the Silverstein Foundation has placed its biggest bets on is a gene-therapy-based company called Prevail Therapeutics. This targeted, patient-driven approach has enabled the company to operate with lightning speed. In just 19 months Prevail Therapeutics' lead gene delivery candidate for GBA-Parkinson's went from inception to initial public offering and IND approval (the first crucial regulatory barrier to cross in clinical drug development). The proposed therapy is among the most promising in all of neurology and is derived from an understanding echoed in this book, that "cures" are only going to come by targeting specific, biologically defined subsets of disease.

Aligning Science Across Parkinson's (ASAP)

Backed by a long-term commitment from the Sergey Brin Family Foundation, ASAP's mandate is to foster collaboration and to direct resources toward better understanding the roots of Parkinson's disease, with the goal of supporting downstream translational efforts.

Sergey Brin's commitment to this cause is very personal. His mother has been living with the disease for nearly 20 years, and he himself is a carrier of a genetic variation associated with Parkinson's (*LRRK2* G2019S). He has long been a prominent supporter of Parkinson's research but now seems ready to take a bold step forward in his commitment through this initiative, which will allocate financial resources to significantly enlarge the basic science effort currently led by government and private foundations.

ASAP is focusing its research efforts within three broad thematic areas, including (1) the biology of PD-associated genetics, (2) neuro-immune interactions, and (3) circuitry and brain–body interactions. The effort will also investigate the pre-symptomatic development of the disease across all three of these research domains in an effort to identify predictive biomarkers and potentially lead to preventative interventions. As of early 2020, ASAP was accepting applications for an initial round of awards of up to $9 million USD over three years to support multidisciplinary research teams working in the first two thematic areas.

In May of 2018 the group held a meeting inviting over 50 Parkinson's experts from around the world to discuss what this roadmap should look like. I was lucky enough to be in attendance, after which Randy Schekman, chair of ASAP and nobel laureate, penned this letter which he asked me to share with the Parkinson's community about this endeavor:

Dear Friends in the PD community,

As you have heard from Ben, the Sergey Brin Family Foundation has had a significant commitment to funding Parkinson's research. Recently this effort has extended to the development of a program on the discovery of how PD begins and spreads to the brain and beyond. Sergey's mother has a genetic form of PD which he inherited, and his former wife, Anne, started and sustains a deep involvement in the company 23andMe, a genetic testing service that you may have used to help identify the numerous genetic forms of PD. Sergey is committed to helping to conquer this disease that we all live with.

I am a basic scientist and have devoted my career to understanding how cells manufacture and export certain protein molecules. We now know that at least one genetic form of PD, the one that afflicts the Brin family, targets an enzyme that acts on a protein my lab discovered almost 40 years ago. Basic research has the power to uncover the secrets of nature that ultimately lead to the cures we seek for the clinic.

But my connection to PD is even more personal as my wife of 44 years died having suffered with PD for the past 20+ years.

After my wife died last year, George Pavlov, CEO of Bayshore Global Management, asked me to Chair the committee looking into a funding mechanism in support of PD research and I jumped at the opportunity to turn my grief into something positive. We just concluded an important meeting of key brain and PD scientists, and patient advocates, Ben included, where we discussed and occasionally argued about the highest priorities for this important work going forward. We reviewed the many avenues of progress on early symptoms of the disease, and the role of genetics, the immune system and brain networks in the progression of PD. Over the next months we will meet with other key funding agencies to map out a blueprint for the Brin Foundation effort to define the most important research goals and how to organize a collaborative effort to make meaningful progress.

I am committed to this program and promise you that my colleagues and I will deploy the power of basic science to discover the insights needed to develop more effective treatments and ultimately cures for the scourge of PD. In the meantime, you can help by attending to the habits of body and mind that are known to delay the progression of PD. Among these habits are a nutritious diet, regular exercise, and active engagement to stretch your brain by reading and communication with others.

I wish you well and ask that you stay tuned as our efforts go forward.

Randy Schekman

University Professor
University of California, Berkeley
Chair, Aligning Science Across Parkinson's (ASAP) Initiative

The Chan Zuckerberg Initiative (CZI)

CZI is the creation of Dr. Priscilla Chan and Mark Zuckerberg. And while the "Z" in CZI may be what gives the group its substantial backing (and adds a Facebook-sized elephant to discussions about it), it is the "C" that is the driving force spurring it forward.

CZI seems to have been born out of a very genuine and abiding moral obligation the couple feels to do good with the unique position they find themselves in. And CZI has the potential to do *a lot* of good – the couple has promised to give to it 99% of a net worth currently valued at $60 billion.

However, the group has attracted some doubt and cynicism fed by rumors of grandiose aims like "cure all disease." But the actual stated goal of CZI Science is a bit more reasonable: "Support the science and technology that will make it possible to cure, prevent, or manage all diseases by the end of the century."[170]

In fact, many of the guiding principles that form CZI's approach to tackling disease resonate with many of the core assertions in this book: a belief that each neurodegenerative disease is not one but hundreds of diseases, the need to break down the silos dividing medical research, the broad search for new mechanisms that trigger and drive disease progression, as well as a commitment to open science.

One of the most ambitious and potentially most impactful projects that CZI has embarked on in its mission to stomp out all disease is the creation of the human cell atlas. A giant collaborative endeavor with labs around the world to map all 37 trillion cells in the human body:

> *The Human Cell Atlas (HCA) is a global collaboration to map and characterize all cells in a healthy human body: cell types, numbers, locations, relationships, and molecular components. It will require advances in single-cell RNA sequencing, image-based transcriptomics and proteomics, tissue handling protocols, data analysis, and more. Once complete, it will be a fundamental resource for scientists, allowing them to better understand how healthy cells work, and what goes wrong when disease strikes.*[171]

Parkinson's disease has been with us ever since we started living long enough for it to develop. Accounts of the disease date as far back as the fifth millennium BC,[172] giving us a minimum of 7,000 years of humans experiencing the steady decline that this disease brings. Included among those humans are some pretty notable figures, including Roman emperor Tiberius, philosopher Thomas Hobbes, and modern despots Hitler and Mao Ze Dong. (The latter two are especially odd for me to think about, as people diagnosed tend to have a kinship with each other over this rare, shared experience.)

All of which puts people who do get diagnosed in a rather unique position in history. While no one in their right mind would ever choose this fate, the silver lining of a diagnosis is that it provides an opportunity to play a role in forever purging humanity of it.

In any narrative, the big picture is always distorted by the point of view of the characters. That is even more profoundly true when the characters are ourselves. It is difficult, if not impossible, to put aside what is happening to us as individuals and our families and connect instead to the larger story. People suffering with disease are well within their right to say, "Who cares about this moment in history. How does any of that help me today?"

Well, it doesn't. It isn't going to help you today, or tomorrow or the day after that. But it does add a little credibility to a phrase people diagnosed often hear, "Now is the best time in history to get diagnosed with Parkinson's." I count myself lucky that of all the generations of people to get this disease, I have a chance of being part of the one that ends it. That has given me the resolve to embrace the daily grind that this disease imposes and do what I can to push research forward so that I have a chance to be among the last generation to know what Parkinson's disease was like.

And when that doesn't work just remember the words of one of the greatest philosophers of our time.

All we have to decide is what to do with the time that is given us.
Gandalf, from J.R.R. Tolkien, *The Fellowship of the Ring*

Epilogue
"When Will We Have a Cure for Parkinson's Disease?"

A decade ago one of my colleagues was asked at a conference, "When will we have a cure for Parkinson's disease?"

"It could happen at any time," he replied. "It could happen next year. It could happen in 10 years. It could happen tomorrow."

My colleague's optimism was well-founded. Talented researchers were hard at work in laboratories throughout the world, and money was pouring in from governments, the pharmaceutical industry, and foundations large and small. The Michael J. Fox Foundation had become a muscular force that was determined to take down this progressive, degenerative disease.

Even better, we knew the targets we were aiming for (or so we thought). Parkinson's disease was caused by abnormal aggregation of proteins in certain parts of the brain, called Lewy bodies, and the loss of brain cells that produced dopamine in a small part of the brain called the substantia nigra.

But after a global investment of over $100 billion, our optimism is tempered. We have no cure to celebrate. Worldwide, 7 to 10 million people suffer from Parkinson's. In the United States, about one million are thought to have Parkinson's, more than those affected by multiple sclerosis, muscular dystrophy and ALS (Lou Gehrig's disease) combined. The cost of Parkinson's in the United States, including treatment and lost productivity, is an estimated $52 billion per year.

Every day people suffering from tremor, slowness, stiffness and balance problems come to us for care. We manage their symptoms with medication ($2,500 per year) or surgery ($100,000), but these are temporary fixes. We have yet to find an effective therapy that slows or modifies the steady march of disability.

It is time to rethink our approach.

We have spent decades explaining the failures of clinical and surgical trials to slow the disease by pointing to shortcomings on technical issues or assuming that we need to study people at earlier and earlier stages. At the same time, we have not questioned the target of those trials. Overwhelming evidence suggests that Parkinson's is actually a syndrome, a group of symptoms that cluster together but have different causes. To make matters more complicated, not all patients have all of these symptoms. And if there are many types of Parkinson's disease, one therapy cannot cure them all.

It is time for the field of neurodegenerative diseases to take a lesson from other fields of medicine and embrace precision medicine – the matching of treatments to biological disease subtypes and the rational use of a multidrug approach for each. The treatment of a patient with breast cancer, for instance, cannot be determined until genetic mutations are identified and receptors are tested. Curing a child with leukemia would not be possible without the ability to use two or more chemotherapy drugs.

Understanding Parkinson's *diseases* according to their molecular subtypes is to see the individual trees in the forest. To see that each subtype requires a different treatment, or even a combination of treatments. To see that one or more of these subtypes may cause symptoms characteristic of both Parkinson's and Alzheimer's diseases. To begin to rethink autopsy studies that have found a high incidence of concurrent Parkinson's and Alzheimer's pathologies in certain groups of patients. And to start the hard work of finding precise biomarkers that will enable us to finally properly define the various subtypes of Parkinson's.

It is humbling to report that, after all these years, we have biomarkers for only a few rare genetic forms of Parkinson's, but none for the subtypes that afflict the vast majority of patients. The field has erred by trying to attach biomarkers to symptoms in patients who already have been diagnosed as having Parkinson's. It is the reverse model – biomarker first, diagnostic subtyping second – that may best inform clinical trials that test new therapies. Because we have used a one-size-fits-all approach to research, assembling clinical trials for all patients rather than for molecular subtypes, we have seen the failure of dozens of trials of promising treatments over the past three decades.

We can only acquire true biomarkers by studying large, aging populations. We need the equivalent of Framingham, the landmark study that revealed high blood pressure and high cholesterol as biomarkers of heart disease. This new approach will require public–private partnerships and data sharing across the globe. It also will require the adoption of flexible clinical trial designs that allow a combination of drug treatments in smaller but well-defined subsets of patients.

Future clinical trials may be conducted not in hundreds or thousands of people with Parkinson's, but rather in dozens of biologically homogeneous patients who share a specific biomarker. In this setting, a cocktail approach may also be needed, as in cancer treatment, to target more than one mechanism of disease.

The transition will require fortitude. We will need to accept that the first proven therapy that protects brain cells may work for fewer than 5% of those assumed to be facing Parkinson's or Alzheimer's. The reward will be our ability to practice true precision medicine for our patients. And it will renew our optimism that diseases of brain aging can someday be slowed and potentially cured – one subtype at a time.

Note Added at Press Time – Reviving LOF

As *Brain Fables* was going through the final stages of publishing we became aware of Dr. Kariem Ezzat's work on the physics of amyloids. In his laboratory at the Karolinska Institute, in Stockholm, he and his team have been examining what happens to proteins as they transform from their soluble to insoluble state (that is, go from being dissolved in the liquids in and around cells to becoming solid objects). Their experiments showed that as the normally soluble protein encounters an abnormal surface, such as a nanoparticle or a virus, referred to as a "nucleating factor", it is forced to aggregate, becoming solid or insoluble; and turns into an amyloid. Many proteins help preserve the integrity of neurons in a soluble state. When they change their shape and become insoluble, they lose their normal function. This loss-of-function (LOF) hypothesis for amyloid has been revived by Dr. Ezzat, based on a "hidden" body of literature, or at least one that has been disregarded by many scientists.

A *gain-of-function* (GOF) hypothesis, whereby the toxicity comes from the accumulation of protein chunks (amyloids) has guided most of the research efforts. This was, in part, because the abnormalities observed when examining brains under a microscope are plaques of amyloid and round bodies of alpha-synuclein. We cannot see the "nucleating factor" or trigger, nor the normal soluble proteins being lost to aggregation.

As discussed in several chapters, therapies for Parkinson's and Alzheimer's have been inspired by the GOF allure, guided by the assumption that aggregated proteins are inherently toxic. Thus, removing them or preventing their aggregation have been viewed as the only viable strategies.

But Dr. Ezzat's research, capitalizing on the overlooked work of others, including that of Sreeganga Chandra, Fredric Manfredsson, Ulrike Müller and Kasper Kepp, suggests that replacing the normal-functioning soluble proteins disappearing into aggregates may restore function and even mitigate the effects of the invisible "nucleating" factors driving the brain into this reactive liquid-to-solid conversion.

The logic appeal of Dr. Ezzat's toxic LOF alternative to the entrenched GOF-driven inspiration for the ongoing antiaggregation efforts in neurodegenerative diseases, is a promising therapeutic frontier. Both of us are brimming with anticipation about its translational potential, whose feasibility will be thoroughly assessed in the months to come.

References

1. Calne DB, Mizuno Y. The neuromythology of Parkinson's Disease. *Parkinsonism Relat Disord*. 2004;10(5):319–322.

2. Postuma RB, Berg D, Stern M, et al. MDS clinical diagnostic criteria for Parkinson's disease. *Mov Disord*. 2015;30 (12):1591–1601.

3. Espay AJ, Schwarzschild MA, Tanner CM, et al. Biomarker-driven phenotyping in Parkinson's disease: a translational missing link in disease-modifying clinical trials. *Mov Disord*. 2017;32(3):319–324.

4. Espay AJ, Vizcarra JA, Marsili L, et al. Revisiting protein aggregation as pathogenic in sporadic Parkinson and Alzheimer diseases. *Neurology*. 2019;92 (7):329–337.

5. Goetz CG. Charcot on Parkinson's disease. *Mov Disord*. 1986;1(1):27–32.

6. Lees AJ. Unresolved issues relating to the shaking palsy on the celebration of James Parkinson's 250th birthday. *Mov Disord*. 2007;22 Suppl 17:S327–334.

7. Langston JW, Palfreman J. *The Case of the Frozen Addicts*. The Netherlands: IOS Press BV; 2014.

8. Langston JW. The MPTP story. *J Parkinsons Dis*. 2017;7(s1):S11–S19.

9. Langston JW, Ballard P, Tetrud JW, Irwin I. Chronic Parkinsonism in humans due to a product of meperidine-analog synthesis. *Science*. 1983;219 (4587):979–980.

10. McCormack AL, Thiruchelvam M, Manning-Bog AB, et al. Environmental risk factors and Parkinson's disease: selective degeneration of nigral dopaminergic neurons caused by the herbicide paraquat. *Neurobiol Dis*. 2002;10 (2):119–127.

11. Golbe LI, Di Iorio G, Bonavita V, Miller DC, Duvoisin RC. A large kindred

with autosomal dominant Parkinson's disease. *Ann Neurol*. 1990;27(3):276–282.

12. Polymeropoulos MH, Higgins JJ, Golbe LI, et al. Mapping of a gene for Parkinson's disease to chromosome 4q21-q23. *Science*. 1996;274(5290):1197–1199.

13. Polymeropoulos MH, Lavedan C, Leroy E, et al. Mutation in the alpha-synuclein gene identified in families with Parkinson's disease. *Science*. 1997;276 (5321):2045–2047.

14. Spillantini MG, Schmidt ML, Lee VM, et al. Alpha-synuclein in Lewy bodies. *Nature*. 1997;388(6645):839–840.

15. Nussbaum RL. The identification of alpha-synuclein as the first Parkinson disease gene. *J Parkinsons Dis*. 2017;7(s1): S43–S49.

16. Braak H, Del Tredici K, Rub U, et al. Staging of brain pathology related to sporadic Parkinson's disease. *Neurobiol Aging*. 2003;24(2):197–211.

17. Shannon KM, Keshavarzian A, Mutlu E, et al. Alpha-synuclein in colonic submucosa in early untreated Parkinson's disease. *Mov Disord*. 2012;27(6):709–715.

18. Shannon KM, Keshavarzian A, Dodiya HB, Jakate S, Kordower JH. Is alpha-synuclein in the colon a biomarker for premotor Parkinson's disease? Evidence from 3 cases. *Mov Disord*. 2012;27(6):716–719.

19. Berg D, Postuma RB, Adler CH, et al. MDS research criteria for prodromal Parkinson's disease. *Mov Disord*. 2015;30 (12):1600–1611.

20. Luk KC, Lee VM. Modeling Lewy pathology propagation in Parkinson's disease. *Parkinsonism Relat Disord*. 2014;20 Suppl 1:S85–S87.

21. Olanow CW, Prusiner SB. Is Parkinson's disease a prion disorder? *Proc Natl Acad Sci U S A*. 2009;106(31):12571–12572.

22. Olanow CW. Do prions cause Parkinson disease?: the evidence accumulates. *Ann Neurol*. 2014;75(3):331–333.

23. Parkkinen L, Kauppinen T, Pirttila T, Autere JM, Alafuzoff I. Alpha-synuclein pathology does not predict extrapyramidal symptoms or dementia. *Ann Neurol*. 2005;57(1):82–91.

24. Mikolaenko I, Pletnikova O, Kawas CH, et al. Alpha-synuclein lesions in normal aging, Parkinson disease, and Alzheimer disease: evidence from the Baltimore Longitudinal Study of Aging (BLSA). *J Neuropathol Exp Neurol*. 2005;64 (2):156–162.

25. Saito Y, Ruberu NN, Sawabe M, et al. Lewy body-related alpha-synucleinopathy in aging. *J Neuropathol Exp Neurol*. 2004;63 (7):742–749.

26. Ding ZT, Wang Y, Jiang YP, et al. Characteristics of alpha-synucleinopathy in centenarians. *Acta Neuropathol*. 2006;111(5):450–458.

27. Burke RE, Dauer WT, Vonsattel JP. A critical evaluation of the Braak staging scheme for Parkinson's disease. *Ann Neurol*. 2008;64(5):485–491.

28. Jellinger KA. A critical reappraisal of current staging of Lewy-related pathology in human brain. *Acta Neuropathol*. 2008;116(1):1–16.

29. Zaccai J, Brayne C, McKeith I, Matthews F, Ince PG. Patterns and stages of alpha-synucleinopathy: relevance in a population-based cohort. *Neurology*. 2008;70(13):1042–1048.

30. Fujita KA, Ostaszewski M, Matsuoka Y, et al. Integrating pathways of Parkinson's disease in a molecular interaction map. *Mol Neurobiol*. 2014;49(1):88–102.

31. Nalls MA, Blauwendraat C, Vallerga CL, et al. Identification of novel risk loci, causal insights, and heritable risk for Parkinson's disease: a meta-analysis of genome-wide association studies. *Lancet Neurol*. 2019;18 (12):1091–1102.

32. Iwaki H, Blauwendraat C, Leonard HL, et al. Genomewide association study of

Parkinson's disease clinical biomarkers in 12 longitudinal patients' cohorts. *Mov Disord*. 2019;34(12):1839–1850.

33. Espay AJ, Brundin P, Lang AE. Precision medicine for disease modification in Parkinson disease. *Nat Rev Neurol*. 2017;13 (2):119–126.

34. Crick F. Central dogma of molecular biology. *Nature*. 1970;227(5258):561–563.

35. Osler W. *The Principles and Practice of Medicine*. NY: Appleton; 1892.

36. Grocott MP. Integrative physiology and systems biology: reductionism, emergence and causality. *Extrem Physiol Med*. 2013;2(1):9.

37. Espay AJ, Lang AE. Parkinson diseases in the 2020s and beyond: replacing clinico-pathologic convergence with systems biology divergence. *J Parkinsons Dis*. 2018;8(s1):S59–S64.

38. Espay AJ. The final nail in the coffin of disease modification for dopaminergic therapies: the LEAP Trial. *JAMA Neurol*. 2019;76(7):747–748.

39. Fahn S, Oakes D, Shoulson I, et al. Levodopa and the progression of Parkinson's disease. *N Engl J Med*. 2004;351 (24):2498–2508.

40. Verschuur CVM, Suwijn SR, Boel JA, et al. Randomized delayed-start trial of levodopa in Parkinson's Disease. *N Engl J Med*. 2019;380(4):315–324.

41. Zetusky WJ, Jankovic J, Pirozzolo FJ. The heterogeneity of Parkinson's disease: clinical and prognostic implications. *Neurology*. 1985;35(4):522–526.

42. Simuni T, Caspell-Garcia C, Coffey C, et al. How stable are Parkinson's disease subtypes in de novo patients: analysis of the PPMI cohort? *Parkinsonism Relat Disord*. 2016;28:62–67.

43. Eisinger RS, Hess CW, Martinez-Ramirez D, et al. Motor subtype changes in early Parkinson's disease. *Parkinsonism Relat Disord*. 2017;43:67–72.

44. Marras C, Lang A. Parkinson's disease subtypes: lost in translation? *J Neurol*

Neurosurg Psychiatry. 2013;84 (4):409–415.

45. Mestre TA, Eberly S, Tanner C, et al. Reproducibility of data-driven Parkinson's disease subtypes for clinical research. *Parkinsonism Relat Disord.* 2018;56:102–106.

46. Fereshtehnejad SM, Zeighami Y, Dagher A, Postuma RB. Clinical criteria for subtyping Parkinson's disease: biomarkers and longitudinal progression. *Brain.* 2017;140(7):1959–1976.

47. De Pablo-Fernandez E, Lees AJ, Holton JL, Warner TT. Prognosis and neuropathologic correlation of clinical subtypes of Parkinson disease. *JAMA Neurol.* 2019;76(4):470–479.

48. Espay AJ, Marras C. Clinical Parkinson disease subtyping does not predict pathology. *Nat Rev Neurol.* 2019;15 (4):189–190.

49. Sorensen AA, Weedon D. Productivity and impact of the top 100 cited Parkinson's disease investigators since 1985. *J Parkinsons Dis.* 2011;1(1):3–13.

50. Buchman AS, Yu L, Wilson RS, et al. Progressive parkinsonism in older adults is related to the burden of mixed brain pathologies. *Neurology.* 2019;92(16): e1821–e1830.

51. Perl DP, Olanow CW, Calne D. Alzheimer's disease and Parkinson's disease: distinct entities or extremes of a spectrum of neurodegeneration? *Ann Neurol.* 1998;44(3 Suppl 1):S19–S31.

52. Irwin DJ, Grossman M, Weintraub D, et al. Neuropathological and genetic correlates of survival and dementia onset in synucleinopathies: a retrospective analysis. *Lancet Neurol.* 2017;16(1):55–65.

53. McKeith IG, Dickson DW, Lowe J, et al. Diagnosis and management of dementia with Lewy bodies: third report of the DLB Consortium. *Neurology.* 2005;65 (12):1863–1872.

54. Devine MJ, Gwinn K, Singleton A, Hardy J. Parkinson's disease and alpha-synuclein expression. *Mov Disord.* 2011;26 (12):2160–2168.

55. Garcia-Ruiz PJ, Espay AJ. Parkinson disease: an evolutionary perspective. *Front Neurol.* 2017;8:157.

56. Ko WKD, Bezard E. Experimental animal models of Parkinson's disease: a transition from assessing symptomatology to alpha-synuclein targeted disease modification. *Exp Neurol.* 2017;298(Pt B):172–179.

57. Buttner S, Broeskamp F, Sommer C, et al. Spermidine protects against alpha-synuclein neurotoxicity. *Cell Cycle* 2014;13(24):3903–3908.

58. Bergstrom AL, Kallunki P, Fog K. Development of passive immunotherapies for synucleinopathies. *Mov Disord.* 2016;31 (2):203–213.

59. Fedak KM, Bernal A, Capshaw ZA, Gross S. Applying the Bradford Hill criteria in the 21st century: how data integration has changed causal inference in molecular epidemiology. *Emerg Themes Epidemiol.* 2015;12:14.

60. Hill AB. The environment and disease: association or causation? 1965. *J R Soc Med.* 2015;108(1):32–37.

61. Janec E, Burke RE. Naturally occurring cell death during postnatal development of the substantia nigra pars compacta of rat. *Mol Cell Neurosci.* 1993;4(1):30–35.

62. Jeon BS, Kholodilov NG, Oo TF, et al. Activation of caspase-3 in developmental models of programmed cell death in neurons of the substantia nigra. *J Neurochem.* 1999;73(1):322–333.

63. Kholodilov NG, Neystat M, Oo TF, et al. Increased expression of rat synuclein in the substantia nigra pars compacta identified by mRNA differential display in a model of developmental target injury. *J Neurochem.* 1999;73(6):2586–2599.

64. Kholodilov NG, Oo TF, Burke RE. Synuclein expression is decreased in rat substantia nigra following induction of apoptosis by intrastriatal 6-hydroxydopamine. *Neurosci Lett.* 1999;275(2):105–108.

65. Stefanis L, Kholodilov N, Rideout HJ, Burke RE, Greene LA. Synuclein-1 is selectively up-regulated in response to

nerve growth factor treatment in PC12 cells. *J Neurochem.* 2001;76 (4):1165–1176.

66. Burke RE. alpha-Synuclein and parkin: coming together of pieces in puzzle of Parkinson's disease. *Lancet.* 2001;358 (9293):1567–1568.

67. Kitada T, Asakawa S, Hattori N, et al. Mutations in the parkin gene cause autosomal recessive juvenile parkinsonism. *Nature.* 1998;392(6676):605–608.

68. Stefanis L, Wang Q, Ou T, et al. Lack of alpha-synuclein does not alter apoptosis of neonatal catecholaminergic neurons. *Eur J Neurosci.* 2004;20(7):1969–1972.

69. Cohen AD, Landau SM, Snitz BE, et al. Fluid and PET biomarkers for amyloid pathology in Alzheimer's disease. *Mol Cell Neurosci.* 2018;97:3-17.

70. Wang J, Dickson DW, Trojanowski JQ, Lee VM. The levels of soluble versus insoluble brain Abeta distinguish Alzheimer's disease from normal and pathologic aging. *Exp Neurol.* 1999;158 (2):328–337.

71. Gilman S, Koller M, Black RS, et al. Clinical effects of Abeta immunization (AN1792) in patients with AD in an interrupted trial. *Neurology.* 2005;64(9):1553–1562.

72. Ostrowitzki S, Lasser RA, Dorflinger E, et al. A phase III randomized trial of gantenerumab in prodromal Alzheimer's disease. *Alzheimers Res Ther.* 2017;9(1):95.

73. Salloway S, Sperling R, Fox NC, et al. Two phase 3 trials of bapineuzumab in mild-to-moderate Alzheimer's disease. *N Engl J Med.* 2014;370(4):322–333.

74. Doody RS, Raman R, Farlow M, et al. A phase 3 trial of semagacestat for treatment of Alzheimer's disease. *N Engl J Med.* 2013;369(4):341–350.

75. Doody RS, Thomas RG, Farlow M, et al. Phase 3 trials of solanezumab for mild-to-moderate Alzheimer's disease. *N Engl J Med.* 2014;370(4):311–321.

76. Honig LS, Vellas B, Woodward M, et al. Trial of solanezumab for mild dementia due to Alzheimer's disease. *N Engl J Med.* 2018;378(4):321–330.

77. Ingelsson M. alpha-Synuclein oligomers-neurotoxic molecules in Parkinson's disease and other Lewy body disorders. *Front Neurosci.* 2016;10:408.

78. Polvikoski T, Sulkava R, Myllykangas L, et al. Prevalence of Alzheimer's disease in very elderly people: a prospective neuropathological study. *Neurology.* 2001;56(12):1690–1696.

79. Markesbery WR, Jicha GA, Liu H, Schmitt FA. Lewy body pathology in normal elderly subjects. *J Neuropathol Exp Neurol.* 2009;68(7):816–822.

80. Balasubramanian AB, Kawas CH, Peltz CB, Brookmeyer R, Corrada MM. Alzheimer disease pathology and longitudinal cognitive performance in the oldest-old with no dementia. *Neurology.* 2012;79 (9):915–921.

81. Silver MH, Newell K, Brady C, Hedley-White ET, Perls TT. Distinguishing between neurodegenerative disease and disease-free aging: correlating neuropsychological evaluations and neuropathological studies in centenarians. *Psychosom Med.* 2002;64(3):493–501.

82. Berlau DJ, Corrada MM, Head E, Kawas CH. APOE epsilon2 is associated with intact cognition but increased Alzheimer pathology in the oldest old. *Neurology.* 2009;72(9):829–834.

83. Kawas CH, Kim RC, Sonnen JA, et al. Multiple pathologies are common and related to dementia in the oldest-old: the 90+ Study. *Neurology.* 2015;85(6):535–542.

84. Latimer CS, Keene CD, Flanagan ME, et al. Resistance to Alzheimer disease neuropathologic changes and apparent cognitive resilience in the Nun and Honolulu-Asia Aging Studies. *J Neuropathol Exp Neurol.* 2017;76 (6):458–466.

85. Robinson JL, Corrada MM, Kovacs GG, et al. Non-Alzheimer's contributions to dementia and cognitive resilience in the 90 + Study. *Acta Neuropathol.* 2018;136 (3):377–388.

86. Ueda K, Fukushima H, Masliah E, et al. Molecular cloning of cDNA encoding an unrecognized component of amyloid in

Alzheimer disease. *Proc Natl Acad Sci U S A*. 1993;90(23):11282–11286.

87. Iwai A, Yoshimoto M, Masliah E, Saitoh T. Non-A beta component of Alzheimer's disease amyloid (NAC) is amyloidogenic. *Biochemistry*. 1995;34(32):10139–10145.

88. Sardi SP, Clarke J, Kinnecom C, et al. CNS expression of glucocerebrosidase corrects alpha-synuclein pathology and memory in a mouse model of Gaucher-related synucleinopathy. *Proc Natl Acad Sci U S A*. 2011;108(29):12101–12106.

89. Parkkinen L, O'Sullivan SS, Collins C, et al. Disentangling the relationship between lewy bodies and nigral neuronal loss in Parkinson's disease. *J Parkinsons Dis*. 2011;1(3):277–286.

90. Hay J, Johnson VE, Smith DH, Stewart W. Chronic traumatic encephalopathy: the neuropathological legacy of traumatic brain injury. *Annu Rev Pathol*. 2016;11:21–45.

91. Farah G, Siwek D, Cummings P. Tau accumulations in the brains of woodpeckers. *PLoS One*. 2018;13(2): e0191526.

92. The Hope List: Parkinson's Therapies in Development. 2019. https://drive.google .com/file/d/1NeSyFA37b9IbUzryRRP-Eqr gScjCRL-3/view. Accessed January 2020.

93. Dumurgier J, Hanseeuw BJ, Hatling FB, et al. Alzheimer's disease biomarkers and future decline in cognitive normal older adults. *J Alzheimers Dis*. 2017;60 (4):1451–1459.

94. Payami H. The emerging science of precision medicine and pharmacogenomics for Parkinson's disease. *Mov Disord*. 2017;32 (8):1139–1146.

95. Mollenhauer B, Caspell-Garcia CJ, Coffey CS, et al. Longitudinal CSF biomarkers in patients with early Parkinson disease and healthy controls. *Neurology*. 2017;89(19):1959-1969.

96. Skillback T, Mattsson N, Hansson K, et al. A novel quantification-driven proteomic strategy identifies an endogenous peptide of pleiotrophin as a new biomarker of Alzheimer's disease. *Sci Rep*. 2017;7 (1):13333.

97. Dumurgier J, Hanseeuw BJ, Hatling FB, et al. Alzheimer's disease biomarkers and future decline in cognitive normal older adults. *J Alzheimers Dis*. 2017;60(4):1451–1459.

98. Postuma RB, Poewe W, Litvan I, et al. Validation of the MDS clinical diagnostic criteria for Parkinson's disease. *Mov Disord*. 2018;33(10):1601–1608.

99. Berg D, Adler CH, Bloem BR, et al. Movement disorder society criteria for clinically established early Parkinson's disease. *Mov Disord*. 2018;33 (10):1643–1646.

100. Kang JH, Mollenhauer B, Coffey CS, et al. CSF biomarkers associated with disease heterogeneity in early Parkinson's disease: the Parkinson's Progression Markers Initiative study. *Acta Neuropathol*. 2016;131(6):935–949.

101. Mollenhauer B, Zimmermann J, Sixel-Doring F, et al. Monitoring of 30 marker candidates in early Parkinson disease as progression markers. *Neurology*. 2016;87 (2):168–177.

102. Thenganatt MA, Jankovic J. Parkinson disease subtypes. *JAMA Neurol*. 2014;71 (4):499–504.

103. Zhu K, van Hilten JJ, Marinus J. Predictors of dementia in Parkinson's disease; findings from a 5-year prospective study using the SCOPA-COG. *Parkinsonism Relat Disord*. 2014;20 (9):980–985.

104. Terrelonge M, Jr., Marder KS, Weintraub D, Alcalay RN. CSF beta-amyloid 1–42 predicts progression to cognitive impairment in newly diagnosed Parkinson disease. *J Mol Neurosci*. 2016;58 (1):88–92.

105. Parnetti L, Gaetani L, Eusebi P, et al. CSF and blood biomarkers for Parkinson's disease. *Lancet Neurol*. 2019;18 (6):573–586.

106. Zhang J, Mattison HA, Liu C, et al. Longitudinal assessment of tau and amyloid beta in cerebrospinal fluid of

Parkinson disease. *Acta Neuropathol.* 2013;126(5):671–682.

107. Parnetti L, Chiasserini D, Persichetti E, et al. Cerebrospinal fluid lysosomal enzymes and alpha-synuclein in Parkinson's disease. *Mov Disord.* 2014;29 (8):1019–1027.

108. Parnetti L, Paciotti S, Eusebi P, et al. Cerebrospinal fluid beta-glucocerebrosidase activity is reduced in Parkinson's disease patients. *Mov Disord.* 2017;32(10):1423–1431.

109. Majbour NK, Vaikath NN, Eusebi P, et al. Longitudinal changes in CSF alpha-synuclein species reflect Parkinson's disease progression. *Mov Disord.* 2016;31 (10):1535–1542.

110. Constantinides VC, Paraskevas GP, Emmanouilidou E, et al. CSF biomarkers beta-amyloid, tau proteins and a-synuclein in the differential diagnosis of Parkinson-plus syndromes. *J Neurol Sci.* 2017;382:91–95.

111. Backstrom DC, Eriksson Domellof M, Linder J, et al. Cerebrospinal fluid patterns and the risk of future dementia in early, incident Parkinson disease. *JAMA Neurol.* 2015;72(10):1175–1182.

112. Chiasserini D, Biscetti L, Eusebi P, et al. Differential role of CSF fatty acid binding protein 3, alpha-synuclein, and Alzheimer's disease core biomarkers in Lewy body disorders and Alzheimer's dementia. *Alzheimers Res Ther.* 2017;9(1):52.

113. Chen-Plotkin AS, Albin R, Alcalay R, et al. Finding useful biomarkers for Parkinson's disease. *Sci Transl Med.* 2018;10(454):pii: eaam6003.

114. Palfreman J. *Brain Storms.* Canada: Harper Collins; 2015.

115. Veronesi U, Saccozzi R, Del Vecchio M, et al. Comparing radical mastectomy with quadrantectomy, axillary dissection, and radiotherapy in patients with small cancers of the breast. *N Engl J Med.* 1981;305(1):6–11.

116. Pharmaceutical Research and Manufacturers of America 2018; http://ph rma-docs.phrma.org/files/dmfile/Alzheim ersSetbacksSteppingStones_FINAL_digita l.pdf. Accessed January 2020.

117. Halsted WS. I. A clinical and histological study of certain adenocarcinomata of the breast: and a brief consideration of the supraclavicular operation and of the results of operations for cancer of the breast from 1889 to 1898 at the Johns Hopkins Hospital. *Ann Surg.* 1898;28 (5):557–576.

118. Veronesi U, Cascinelli N, Mariani L, et al. Twenty-year follow-up of a randomized study comparing breast-conserving surgery with radical mastectomy for early breast cancer. *N Engl J Med.* 2002;347 (16):1227–1232.

119. Malhotra GK, Zhao X, Band H, Band V. Histological, molecular and functional subtypes of breast cancers. *Cancer Biol Ther.* 2010;10(10):955–960.

120. Bianchini G, Balko JM, Mayer IA, Sanders ME, Gianni L. Triple-negative breast cancer: challenges and opportunities of a heterogeneous disease. *Nat Rev Clin Oncol.* 2016;13(11):674–690.

121. The Economist. European countries demand that publicly funded research be free. www.economist.com/science-and-te chnology/2018/09/15/european-coun tries-demand-that-publicly-funded-resea rch-be-free. Accessed January 2020.

122. Gold ER. Should Universities Get Out Of The Patent Business? 2019; www.cigion line.org/articles/should-universities-get-o ut-patent-business. Accessed January 2020.

123. Perry TL, Godin DV, Hansen S. Parkinson's disease: a disorder due to nigral glutathione deficiency? *Neurosci Lett.* 1982;33(3):305–310.

124. Shults CW, Haas RH, Beal MF. A possible role of coenzyme Q10 in the etiology and treatment of Parkinson's disease. *Biofactors.* 1999;9(2–4):267–272.

125. Parain K, Murer MG, Yan Q, et al. Reduced expression of brain-derived neurotrophic factor protein in Parkinson's disease substantia nigra. *Neuroreport.* 1999;10(3):557–561.

126. Hunot S, Bernard V, Faucheux B, et al. Glial cell line-derived neurotrophic factor (GDNF) gene expression in the human brain: a post mortem in situ hybridization study with special reference to Parkinson's disease. *J Neural Transm (Vienna)*. 1996;103(8–9):1043–1052.

127. Beal MF, Oakes D, Shoulson I, et al. A randomized clinical trial of high-dosage coenzyme Q10 in early Parkinson disease: no evidence of benefit. *JAMA Neurol*. 2014;71(5):543–552.

128. Kieburtz K, Tilley BC, Elm JJ, et al. Effect of creatine monohydrate on clinical progression in patients with Parkinson disease: a randomized clinical trial. *JAMA*. 2015;313(6):584–593.

129. The Parkinson Study Group. Effect of deprenyl on the progression of disability in early Parkinson's disease: the Parkinson Study Group. *New Engl J Med*. 1989;321(20):1364–1371.

130. Snow BJ, Rolfe FL, Lockhart MM, et al. A double-blind, placebo-controlled study to assess the mitochondria-targeted antioxidant MitoQ as a disease-modifying therapy in Parkinson's disease. *Mov Disord*. 2010;25(11):1670–1674.

131. Writing Group for the NETiPDI, Kieburtz K, Tilley BC, et al. Effect of creatine monohydrate on clinical progression in patients with Parkinson disease: a randomized clinical trial. *JAMA*. 2015;313(6):584–593.

132. Investigators N-PF-Z. Pioglitazone in early Parkinson's disease: a phase 2, multicentre, double-blind, randomised trial. *Lancet Neurol*. 2015;14(8):795–803.

133. Rascol O, Olanow CW, Brooks D, et al. A 2-year multicenter, placebo-controlled, double-blind, parallel group study of the effect of riluzole on Parkinson's disease progression. *Mov Disord*. 2002;17 (Suppl 5):39.

134. Shults CW. Effect of selegiline (deprenyl) on the progression of disability in early Parkinson's disease: Parkinson Study Group. *Acta Neurol Scand Suppl*. 1993;146:36–42.

135. Parkinson Study Group QE3 Investigtors, Beal MF, Oakes D, et al. A randomized clinical trial of high-dosage coenzyme Q10 in early Parkinson disease: no evidence of benefit. *JAMA Neurol*. 2014;71(5):543–552.

136. Myllyla VV, Sotaniemi KA, Vuorinen JA, Heinonen EH. Selegiline as initial treatment in de novo parkinsonian patients. *Neurology*. 1992;42(2):339–343.

137. Olanow CW, Rascol O, Hauser R, et al. A double-blind, delayed-start trial of rasagiline in Parkinson's disease. *N Engl J Med*. 2009;361(13):1268–1278.

138. Schapira AH, McDermott MP, Barone P, et al. Pramipexole in patients with early Parkinson's disease (PROUD): a randomised delayed-start trial. *Lancet Neurol*. 2013;12(8):747–755.

139. Hauser RA, Lyons KE, McClain T, Carter S, Perlmutter D. Randomized, double-blind, pilot evaluation of intravenous glutathione in Parkinson's disease. *Mov Disord*. 2009;24(7):979–983.

140. Olanow W, Bartus RT, Baumann TL, et al. Gene delivery of neurturin to putamen and substantia nigra in Parkinson disease: a double-blind, randomized, controlled trial. *Ann Neurol*. 2015;78(2):248–257.

141. Lang AE, Gill S, Patel NK, et al. Randomized controlled trial of intraputamenal glial cell line-derived neurotrophic factor infusion in Parkinson disease. *Ann Neurol*. 2006;59(3):459–466.

142. Ribeiro MJ, Stoessl AJ, Brooks D. Evaluation of a potential neurotrophic drug on the progression of Parkinson disease with 18FDOPA. *J Nucl Med*. 2006;50(Suppl. 2):A125.

143. Clinicaltrials.gov. https://clinicaltrials.gov/ct2/show/NCT01060878. Accessed January 2020.

144. NINDS NET-PD Investigators. A randomized, double-blind, futility clinical trial of creatine and minocycline in early Parkinson disease. *Neurology*. 2006;66(5):664–671.

145. GPI 1485 Study Group. GPI 1485, a neuroimmunophilin ligand, fails to alter

disease progression in mild to moderate Parkinson's disease. *Mov Disord.* 2006;21: A1009.

146. Olanow CW, Schapira AH, LeWitt PA, et al. TCH346 as a neuroprotective drug in Parkinson's disease: a double-blind, randomised, controlled trial. *Lancet Neurol.* 2006;5(12):1013–1020.

147. Parkinson Study Group. Mixed lineage kinase inhibitor CEP-1347 fails to delay disability in early Parkinson disease. *Neurology.* 2007;69 (15):1480–1490.

148. Kaiser J. The Alzheimer's gamble. *Science.* 2018;361(6405):838–841.

149. Panza F, Lozupone M, Logroscino G, Imbimbo BP. A critical appraisal of amyloid-beta-targeting therapies for Alzheimer disease. *Nat Rev Neurol.* 2019;15(2):73–88.

150. Knopman DS. Bad news and good news in AD, and how to reconcile them. *Nat Rev Neurol.* 2019;15(2):61–62.

151. Cummings JL, Cohen S, van Dyck CH, et al. ABBY: A phase 2 randomized trial of crenezumab in mild to moderate Alzheimer disease. *Neurology.* 2018;90 (21):e1889–e1897.

152. Egan MF, Kost J, Tariot PN, et al. Randomized trial of verubecestat for mild-to-moderate Alzheimer's disease. *N Engl J Med.* 2018;378(18):1691–1703.

153. Biogen. Biogen Plans Regulatory Filing for Aducanumab in Alzheimer's disease Based on New Analysis of Larger Dataset from Phase 3 Studies. http://investors.bio gen.com/news-releases/news-release-deta ils/biogen-plans-regulatory-filing-aduca numab-alzheimers-disease. Accessed January 2020.

154. Scheuerle A. Limits of the genetic revolution. *Arch Pediatr Adolesc Med.* 2001;155(11):1204–1209.

155. Frisoni GB, Ritchie C, Carrera E, et al. Re-aligning scientific and lay narratives of Alzheimer's disease. *Lancet Neurol.* 2019;18(10):918–919.

156. Kannel WB. Framingham study insights into hypertensive risk of cardiovascular disease. *Hypertens Res.* 1995;18 (3):181–196.

157. Jack CR, Jr., Bennett DA, Blennow K, et al. NIA-AA research framework: toward a biological definition of Alzheimer's disease. *Alzheimers Dement.* 2018;14 (4):535–562.

158. Jack CR, Jr., Therneau TM, Weigand SD, et al. Prevalence of biologically vs clinically defined Alzheimer spectrum entities using the National Institute on Aging-Alzheimer's Association research framework. *JAMA Neurol.* 2019; Jul 15 (Epub ahead of print) (DOI:10.1001/ jamaneurol.2019.1971).

159. Shokri-Kojori E, Wang GJ, Wiers CE, et al. beta-Amyloid accumulation in the human brain after one night of sleep deprivation. *Proc Natl Acad Sci U S A.* 2018;115(17):4483–4488.

160. Xie L, Kang H, Xu Q, et al. Sleep drives metabolite clearance from the adult brain. *Science.* 2013;342(6156):373–377.

161. Riordan JR, Rommens JM, Kerem B, et al. Identification of the cystic fibrosis gene: cloning and characterization of complementary DNA. *Science.* 1989;245 (4922):1066–1073.

162. Flume PA, Liou TG, Borowitz DS, et al. Ivacaftor in subjects with cystic fibrosis who are homozygous for the F508del-CFTR mutation. *Chest.* 2012;142(3):718–724.

163. Accurso FJ, Rowe SM, Clancy JP, et al. Effect of VX-770 in persons with cystic fibrosis and the G551D-CFTR mutation. *N Engl J Med.* 2010;363(21):1991–2003.

164. Ramsey BW, Davies J, McElvaney NG, et al. A CFTR potentiator in patients with cystic fibrosis and the G551D mutation. *N Engl J Med.* 2011;365 (18):1663–1672.

165. Dorsey ER, Sherer T, Okun MS, Bloem BR. The emerging evidence of the Parkinson pandemic. *J Parkinsons Dis.* 2018;8(s1):S3-S8.

166. Brockman JE. *This Idea Must Die: Scientific Theories That Are Blocking Progress.* New York: HarperCollins Publishers; 2015.

167. Cedarbaum JM. Elephants, Parkinson's disease, and proof-of-concept clinical trials. *Mov Disord.* 2018;33(5):697–700.

168. Lang AE, Espay AJ. Disease modification in Parkinson's disease: current approaches, challenges, and future considerations. *Mov Disord.* 2018;33(5):660–677.

169. The Australian Parkinson's Mission. 2019; https://scienceofparkinsons.com/2019/01/30/apm/. Accessed January 2020.

170. Chan Zuckerbert Initiative. 2019; https://chanzuckerberg.com/science/. Accessed January 2020.

171. Chan Zuckerberg Initiative. Human Cell Atlas. https://chanzuckerberg.com/science/programs-resources/humancellatlas/. Accessed January 2020.

172. Raudino F. The Parkinson disease before James Parkinson. *Neurol Sci.* 2012;33(4):945–948.

Index